Endorsement

Judy Ponsford offers wisdom, expertise, and empathy to provide the utmost care for her patients. She has invested this same energy in writing *You, GOD, Hormones, and Health!* In working with Judy, thousands of patients have discovered the individual care that is missing from the typical clinic setting found today. *You, GOD, Hormones, and Health* offers this same level of individual support with a clear road map for restoring your body, mind, and spirit.

Jean Brickell, N.D., CBS, CNC

You, GOD, Hormones, and Health

An Informative and Inspirational Guide to Wellness

Judy Ponsford, BSN, RN, WHNP

WESTBOW
PRESS
A DIVISION OF THOMAS NELSON

Cover Artist: Virginia Popp. Signed prints may be obtained by contacting Judy's office at (303) 805 - 5466. Priced according to size.

WestBow Press books may be ordered through booksellers or by contacting:

WestBow Press
A Division of Thomas Nelson
1663 Liberty Drive
Bloomington, IN 47403
www.westbowpress.com
1-(866) 928-1240

ISBN: 978-1-4497-2942-4 (e)
ISBN: 978-1-4497-2943-1 (sc)
ISBN: 978-1-4497-2944-8 (hc)

Library of Congress Control Number: 2011919055

Printed in the United States of America

WestBow Press rev. date: 4/4/2013

Dedication

For all my clients who said, "Could you *please* write that down?"

To my wonderful husband, Michael, who rolls with the punches when I do *crazy* things like starting a business in a recession or deciding to write a book. I could do none of this without your love, support, and patience.

To my precious family who means the world to me, gives me so much joy, and is always there encouraging, inspiring, praying for me, and supporting my endeavors:

- Rob and Jenn, Chris, Angelina, David, and Lilly Pea
- Dave and Jayla, Jayden, Chaselyn, and Jori Bug
- Shannon, Ginger, and Michaiah
- Mom English (pediatric nurse practitioner, retired), who at eighty-three is still an inspiration to us all with her daily walks and very healthy eating habits.
- Mom Parker (deceased), who was my prayer warrior and would have been so proud. I miss you so much!

Acknowledgments

As with most endeavors in life, writing a book takes the collaborative work of many individuals. Every person who has even looked at or touched this work has placed his or her mark on it in a significant way, and I could not have brought this to completion without their help:

Jean Brickell, ND: Thank you for your endorsement of this book. God blessed me with you, a like-minded practitioner and dear friend to partner with in my business. Priceless!

Brooke Caustrida: Thanks for citing my references for me in a timely manner. It was a chore that was dragging me down. You helped to get me going again!

Jennifer Lundy: My ongoing prayer warrior for my business and this book.

Pollyanna Pastor: Thank you for editing, proofing, and giving me better ideas about wording and phrasing my paragraphs and also for your medical expertise that kept me factual. Your help has been so very valuable to me.

Jayla Ponsford: Thank you so much for helping me edit the book and citing some of my references. Also, thanks for your computer knowledge and help in getting the book formatted correctly.

Michael Ponsford: With all the many hats you wear in our family, thanks also for taking the time to read and proof my book and give me better eyes from a reader's perspective.

Ginger Popp: Thank you to my beautiful daughter and faithful prayer warrior for my business and this project. Your most beautiful artwork was destined and perfectly suited for this book.

Tammy Thomas: Thanks for helping edit and proof the book. Your knowledge and background in nutrition and the body systems is amazing. I truly appreciated your feedback.

Contents

Introduction and Philosophy

Making decisions about health can be very difficult and frustrating at times for many women. Often questions arise concerning particular health subjects, such as hormones, heart health, issues with the thyroid or other body systems and how they interrelate, as well as general health-care concerns. I understand the notion that subjects concerning well-being are just plain confusing at times. There is so much contradictory information available in all forms of media these days, which continually creates uncertainty about who or what to believe. To make matters even more burdensome, the answer(s) for any particular health dilemma is different for each and every woman because of individual body composition, genetics, and the existing level of wellness. Sorting through all of this information can be a daunting task but a necessary and worthy responsibility that I advocate.

After working in women's health for over fifteen years and the field of bioidentical hormones and holistic and integrated health care for over twelve years, I have endeavored to take what I have experienced and believe to be some of the more popular health topics that I sense women often feel confused and unsure about and combine them under one cover. It is my desire for this book to serve as a valuable informative resource on these particular subjects. Also in these pages I have specifically made it my duty to inspire you to grasp the importance of becoming your own advocate when it comes to health matters. If you don't take the initiative to be proactive in such matters, no one else can do it for you. I am likewise confident that this book features practical and preventative health-care measures that, when put into practice, will support vitality and the antiaging process. It is never too late to begin any practice that will improve your health and well-being. Additionally, I am firmly convinced that we are more than just bodies or physical beings. Our spirits play a momentous role in our physical and mental health and the healing process. It is my wish that these pages also provide you with inspirational Scriptures and words that will touch your spirit and help you soar to be all God intended you to be, regardless of where you are in your spiritual life and chronological or biological age.

Because of my very nature and trust in God, I am a naturalist at heart. I believe that if God went to great lengths to create such an amazing and incredible machine that we call our body, we should do our very best to take care of it. Psalm 139:14 says, "For You formed my inward parts; You covered me in my mother's womb. I will praise You, for I am fearfully and wonderfully made; Marvelous are Your works, And that my soul knows very well." And 1 Corinthians 6:19 states, "Do you not know that your body is the temple of the Holy Spirit who is in you, whom you have from God, and you are not your own?" (NIV). I love reading those particular verses because they remind me daily that God did take great care in creating my body, and I am wholly His. Therefore, if we are "fearfully and wonderfully made" by God *and* if our bodies are "holy temples" of the Lord, then shouldn't we put the greatest care and thought into what we do *to* and *with* our bodies?

We know as Christians that one day we will have resurrected bodies that are free from all of the ravages of sin and this fallen earth, and we won't have to be concerned about our health. But think about it: even the risen Christ in His perfect, changed, eternal, resurrected body still carried the scars on His pierced hands, feet, and side from the agony of the cross. My thought is that we need to be very conscientious about how we care for ourselves. To the best of our ability, we should honor our bodies as God's marvelous handiwork and make good decisions concerning what we do *to* and *with* our bodies in terms of health care. I know that on this fallen earth there are no perfect answers, so I am not going to claim I have perfect answers. However, as I stated above, I hope to offer you a resource and guidance in the areas of my expertise and together with you call upon our heavenly Father to help you choose that which is good and right in your particular circumstance(s).

When I first began practicing as a women's health nurse practitioner, one of the first things I did was sit down and write a business statement to which I dedicated myself concerning my practice and the treatment of my clients. It goes something like this: "I promise to treat each woman I serve as though I were treating myself, to the best of my ability; to see her as God's child and honor the potential she can attain here on this earth; and to give her the time, information, and attention she deserves as God's creation." I still read this to myself often. This statement helps me to stay centered on the purpose for which I became a practitioner. It also helps me to stay focused on my clients and the role I play in each of their lives. For all of my clients, I see myself as serving them in the ministry of health and healing. I do not and will not practice or suggest to clients anything or any kind of treatment that I would not consider doing myself in their particular situation. Though I may never meet most of you (my readers) face to face, this desire still holds true within the writings of this book. I want each of you to know that I hold your interest to the highest level and pray that you will do the same for your own body as you prayerfully make health-care decisions based on godly wisdom.

Furthermore, I consider listening to be a very important element in health care. I try my best to practice that characteristic for each of my patients. I once read that if you listen to patients long enough, they will tell you their correct diagnoses. If you continue to listen to them even longer, they will tell you what should be done to treat them. Listening in the health-care field has become a lost art. Most practitioners do not have the time to listen to their clients long enough to treat them properly. Short visits of ten to fifteen minutes are common. I pray that I will *listen* long and intently enough to each patient in which I come into contact that I will be able to determine the exact root of the problem(s) and implement the correct treatment(s). Finding a provider that is a good listener is essential in quality health care.

I also believe that a really good health-care provider is an educator. Prior to my nursing career, I began my studies in education. Secondary to that background and my love for teaching, I truly enjoy taking small groups of women and teaching them about hormones and other health matters. I strive to educate each client as much as possible on her particular situation(s) as they arise. However, I have never believed that it is the total responsibility of the provider to *spoon-feed* the patient on all health-care matters. I always encourage my patients to ask questions, seek out information, read, and educate themselves on their relevant subjects of health. I have learned the most motivated and compliant patients are those who are informed on the subject that is being discussed. The more informed they are, the better I can partner with them to implement what we believe together to be the most effective and best regimen/treatment possible to improve their condition and overall general health.

No, health education is not just the provider's responsibility; it is imperative for the patient too. However, it is the responsibility of providers to see that patients have as much information imparted to them as is possible that relates to their condition(s). One-on-one teaching during the appointment gives me as a provider confidence that not only am I doing the best I can do, but also that my client and I, with the Father in heaven, are partners in their health care. I earnestly believe I am supposed to be a coworker with Christ. I know that only Christ can give deliverance from sin, but as His coworker in the health-care field, I can be His vessel in *deliverance from* and *prevention of* disease in this life.

When it comes to your spiritual life, that is something you must seek. There are passages in the Scriptures that talk about God *hiding* Himself from us. Isaiah 45:15 says, "Truly you are a God who hides Himself, O God and Savior of Israel." You just read above that He is our Creator, and we are the temples in which He resides. Why would He want to hide from us? Upon creation, God issued each and every one of us that thing we call a *free will*. He never forces Himself on anyone but delights in our relationship with and pursuit of Him and His ways. In other words, Christ is the lover of our soul. If we choose to love Him back, it is not enough to just say, "I choose You." The desire in our hearts to know Him should put us into action to study and learn His Word and His ways so we may know what pleases Him and eventually develop that intimate relationship with Him that our hearts so long for. Thus, I firmly believe that this is how Christ also wants us to pursue all the other important things and areas in our life. If we have questions and concerns about anything (health-wise), we need to spring into action and begin searching out information from reliable sources, go to the Father in prayer, and search the Scriptures. At some point, we can trust that God *will* help us emerge with a decision that we personally own, knowing the decision and conclusion we have made will honor God in us.

And though He desires that we search for Him and His righteous ways, He is *not* a God of confusion. He *will* reveal all things to those

God made a world in which we have the freedom to choose, knowing that many would reject Him and a few would choose to give their affections in worship to the One who made it all. God would rather have the meaningful worship of a few rather than the robotic worship of the masses. Nobody wants coerced affection least of all God. Genuine worship and love from the souls of a few—that's the choice God made.

—James MacDonald
Downpour

God loves the hide-and-seek of life because it requires faith. Faith is what enables us to endure, believe, and trust in what we can't see.

—Bob Coy
Dreamality

who truly seek after Him. Second Timothy 2:15 says, "Study to show thyself approved, a workman that needs not to be ashamed, rightly dividing the word of truth." John 16:13 declares, "Howbeit when He, the spirit of truth, is come, He will guide you into all truth." If we really want something, then we must seek after it. I thoroughly understand that there will be those emergency situations in which we do not have that valued thing called *time* on our side, and taking precious time to make a particular decision about our health may not be possible. However, in terms of preventative health care, let us not take this responsibility lightly.

As you embark on reading the rest of this book, I pray that you keep in mind that improving the quality of your health is my greatest desire. To the best of my ability, I have studied, researched, practiced, and sought after truth in these areas in which I am writing. I honestly believe that you can take my experience and knowledge about these solid health principles presented to you in this book and use them to improve your overall general health and *prevent* disease. Some of the ideas may be different than you have encountered before or to some degree away from mainstream thinking, but I believe the way our culture relates to health and wellness is inadequate, to say the least. It is time for a major paradigm shift in how we approach the care of our bodies as well as our health-care system. I am here to give you a gentle shove in that direction. Enjoy, and good health!

Hold on to instruction, do not let it go, guard it well, for it is your life.

Proverbs 4:13

Prayer: Lord, we all need to seek instruction, but remind us that we should first pray and then seek it from sources that are based on your principles.

Amen

Chapter 1

Hormones

I will begin with the subject of hormone therapy because hormones have been my specialty for over twelve years. Not only have I worked with hundreds of women over the past years helping to balance their hormones, but I too have walked that l-o-n-g road of perimenopause and now menopause. Most of what I have to say I have experienced. It may not be to the degree that many of my clients over the years have experienced (or even many of you), but I definitely can say that I have walked in those shoes. Personal and clinical experience and the ongoing education that maintains my certification as a hormone specialist largely provides the sum total of my knowledge in this area.

The subject of hormones is complicated. To further complicate the issue, women differ by body composition and their level of overall general health. Using hormones should not be taken lightly and requires the assistance of someone with skill and expertise. Bioidentical hormone replacement therapy (BHRT) receives my highest recommendation. I do not advocate the use of synthetic hormones (i.e., hormones that are not bioidentical in their chemical structure when compared to what the body does or would naturally make). If you want to know the long-term effects of synthetic hormones, you can Google the subject and read the results of different trial arms of the Women's Health Initiative (WHI) from June 2002 that demonstrate the many adverse effects of long-term treatment with both synthetic estrogens and progestins (synthetic progesterone). When I speak about hormones in this book, please be aware that I will be directly referring to BHRT unless I say otherwise. Trying to make synthetic and bioidentical hormones equal or interchangeable is just not possible. It is like saying apples are oranges, and you just cannot do that. I only recommend, prescribe, and personally take BHRT.

To date, there are a number of books available on the subject of bioidentical hormones. Suzanne Sommers' *The Sexy Years*, Christiane Northrop MD's *The Wisdom of Menopause,* and John Lee MD's *What Your Doctor May Not Tell You About Menopause* are good examples. All of these books have helped so many women and brought to light the fact that different options do exist. As a result of the fact that pharmaceutical companies have the money to advertise and research to a much greater degree than anyone else, these other options in the way of hormones have not been widely made known in the past. We owe much of the information and knowledge about additional hormone options and BHRT to people like the authors mentioned above. Therefore, I am not trying to duplicate all the information in those books. What I would like to focus on in this chapter, though, are questions that may arise in your own mind about those options. I will provide you with facts based on the guidance of sound medical advisors, authors, and researchers who do not lend themselves greatly to the pharmaceutical companies. I will also offer inspirational words to encourage you when these questions do arise in your life.

Why should you even consider taking BHRT?

First, let us begin with a little bit of a physiology lesson. The reproductive cycle can be studied in a number of books, so I do not plan to review that here. However, let us consider what happens when the majority of women experience hormonal changes. There is no set age for this. Symptoms of perimenopause can begin in the mid to late thirties or possibly younger, depending on a number of factors, such as ovarian failure, cystic ovaries, environmental factors, and a person's individual health status, diet, and number and/or kind of pelvic surgeries. The fact is, when you begin having anovulatory (no egg or ovum is released) cycles, regardless of the reason or age, progesterone levels decrease, and thus, estrogen becomes dominant. Low progesterone creates estrogen dominance or an imbalance in the progesterone-to-estrogen ratio. This is basically what I call perimenopause. Mild symptoms may occur in the beginning, but as the number of anovulatory cycles increases, the situation can worsen. Symptoms may begin with occasional restless nights, premenstrual syndrome (PMS) that is worse than is normal, mild headaches, an increase in fatigue, and slightly heavier and/or crampier periods. As time goes on, the same symptoms can become even more severe, with added problems such as irregular or excessive bleeding.

When the ovaries completely shut down and there are no viable follicles left to produce estrogen, bleeding will cease (menopause) because there is neither estrogen to build a uterine lining nor progesterone to decidualize (release) the uterine lining, even if there were a remnant lining remaining. Once estrogen and progesterone have stopped being produced by the ovaries altogether, the adrenal glands become the primary source of these hormones. Although you will read more about the adrenals in chapter 5, I feel it is necessary to include some pertinent information here and explain how closely hormones relate to the adrenal system.

It is common scientific knowledge that both estrogen and progesterone are used in hundreds of biochemical and enzymatic reactions in the female body for optimal functioning. Since the ovaries are unable to produce the hormones during menopause, the adrenal glands must now take on this duty. That may not be a problem for a woman whose adrenal glands are healthy and strong in the short-term. However, the adrenal glands have many functions, and the added stress of having to produce hormones as well can *begin to* or *eventually will* cause adrenal fatigue.

Today's lifestyles are generally stressful on the adrenal system for the average woman secondary to the high cortisol (the adrenal stress hormone) levels, which stress induces. By the time one reaches menopause, the added stress of having to produce hormones as well will typically send the adrenals into a hypo-functioning (low-functioning) state to some degree. I find that adding progesterone in early perimenopause and then adding the estrogen component at menopause supports the adrenal glands and prevents further hypoadrenia (low adrenal function).

It is a difficult task to fully express the importance of the adrenal system. There have been volumes of books written on this subject and how the adrenal system relates to every function in the body. This system is quite complicated; however, I do believe from experience, both

A part can never be well unless the whole is well.

—Plato

Health is a state of complete harmony of the body, mind, and spirit. When one is free from physical disabilities and mental distractions, the gates of the soul open.

—B. K. S. Iyengar

personally and clinically, that I have grasped the importance of taking care of the adrenals. I have seen the sometimes slow but eventually devastating effects of low hormone levels on the adrenal system. The adrenal system and its function is a very necessary component when deciding on BHRT. I will refer to the adrenal system repeatedly in this book because as I see it, all roads or aspects of our health lead to the adrenal glands. James L. Wilson writes in *Adrenal Fatigue, The 21ˢᵗ Century Stress Syndrome:*

> With adrenal fatigue, the sex hormone levels often fall because your adrenal glands are not able to manufacture adequate levels of hormones. One function that sex hormones serve is to act as anti-oxidants that help prevent the oxidative damage caused by cortisol. So the lower the sex hormones, the more damage there is to tissues, especially when you are under stress. This oxidative damage is one of the key factors in rapid aging.[1]

Essentially, taking or using BHRT has antiaging effects. And as I have found in my practice, BHRT, although not all inclusive, is one of several important ways to support the adrenal glands, ward off disease processes, and slow the aging process.

Diana Schwarzbein, MD, is a leading authority on the adrenal system. She has written several books on the subject and has personally walked the path of severe adrenal burnout and eventual rebuilding. One of her books, *The Schwarzbein Principle II,* covers the subject of the adrenal system and recommends hormone replacement therapy to support the adrenals, if deficiency exists.

She says something that I think you will find very interesting. The major hormones like adrenaline, cortisol, and insulin are essential for life. If one of these major hormones is missing, illness occurs quickly, and you will not live very long; therefore, there should be (and usually is) no controversy about whether or not these hormones should be replaced.

However, since the minor hormones, such as estradiol, progesterone, testosterone, and DHEA-Sulfate, do not cause quite as rapid a decline in health, there always seems to be a ruckus surrounding them. She asserts that the lack of the minor hormones will also cause death, but because it may come ten to fifteen years later, typically no one is going to attribute the demise to the lack of those minor hormones. They *all* play a crucial role in health and longevity, and it is extremely important that both the major and minor hormones be kept in balance. She further emphasizes that hormones control regeneration in the body; when your hormones are not balanced, your body's ability to regenerate is compromised.[2]

When you truly understand this concept of how the adrenals affect *every* system in the body, as we talked about previously, then you can grasp the notion of how this theory can be true. Once you lose your hormones, believe me, you are on a freight train headed downhill, and there is no stopping it! What you do to enhance the functioning of your adrenal system determines how fast that train is going to go. Again, BHRT can be a very important piece of the puzzle that supports adrenal function, your overall general health, and how fast you are going to age (or die, for that matter).

I realize that history shows there are a few women on both ends of the hormone spectrum. Some will experience menopause with few problems, take no hormone therapy, and live a very long and healthy life. Some, on the other hand, will have horrible symptoms and will not get the results they want (even from BHRT), and their health will continue to decline. Then there are the rest of us right in the middle who most likely will have good results from BHRT. What I have seen clinically for this majority certainly favors BHRT as a good treatment option for helping to preserve the adrenals as well as being beneficial for overall good physical and mental health.

Why is progesterone deficiency and/or estrogen dominance harmful?

Progesterone deficiency and estrogen dominance are one and the same (so to speak) in terms of the problems this imbalance may cause. As you read above, anovulatory cycles mark the beginning of perimenopause as progesterone levels decline. Although estrogen levels do not go up, the ratio of progesterone to estrogen is very low; thus, there is estrogen dominance. The progesterone to estrogen (P:E) ratio should be between two hundred to one and three hundred to one on a saliva test.[3] For those of you who test your hormones by serum blood, see Appendix IV to calculate your P:E ratio. As a woman progresses through a life span of hormone cycles, this ratio becomes lower and lower (i.e., of progesterone to estrogen). Eventually in menopause this ratio may improve to some degree because estrogen levels also decline. However, the imbalance is doing or has already done its harm.

There are many conditions in which this state of low progesterone and estrogen dominance are associated. Low progesterone and estrogen dominance have been associated with endometriosis, the growth of uterine fibroids, breast pain, fibrocystic breasts, thyroid dysfunction, osteoporosis (yes, I said osteoporosis, so read on), migraine headaches, fatigue, low libido, depression, heavy/clotty/crampy menstrual cycles, allergies, breast cancer, foggy thinking, and more. Let me cover some of these areas in a little more detail.

Endometriosis: This is a very painful condition that develops when endometrial cells (cells that line the uterus) implant and form colonies outside of the uterus in the pelvic cavity. These endometrial implants can attach to the ovaries, fallopian tubes, intestines, bladder, and any other organ. These endometrial cells begin to grow, multiply, fill up with blood, and bleed into the surrounding areas and tissues during menstruation. Because the blood has nowhere to go, it causes inflammation, scarring and adhesions, and a great deal of pain and suffering for its victims.[4] Although curing endometriosis is difficult, it has long been known that progesterone is the hormone of choice to try and reduce some of the inflammation and pain. Many providers will put their clients on birth control pills (synthetic hormones), particularly progestin-only pills, because they know that the progestin will oppose the estrogenic effects of these endometrial cell implants. Instead of offering birth control pills to clients seeking my advice, I prefer to offer and prescribe bioidentical progesterone to oppose the estrogen and help alleviate the pain.

Uterine Fibroids: These are noncancerous growths that usually shrink during menopause when estrogen levels drop. However, long before that, an imbalance in hormones or estrogen dominance can and will fuel the growth of these tumors, the number-one reason for hysterectomies, especially symptomatic fibroids causing pain and bleeding. Few women are given the choice of a therapeutic trial of bioidentical progesterone as an option to help oppose the estrogen effect, slow the growth, and at least keep these tumors at bay until menopause,

And a woman was there who had been crippled by a spirit for eighteen years. She was bent over and could not straighten up at all. When Jesus saw her, he called her forward and said to her, "Woman, you are set free from your infirmity."

—Luke 13:11–13

At first when I thought about His calling her, I thought, "How rude to call her." Why didn't He speak the word and heal her in her seat. Perhaps God wants to see us moving toward Him. We need to invest in our own deliverance. We will bring a testimony out of a test. I also believe that someone else there had problems. When we can see someone else overcoming a handicap, it helps us to overcome.

—T. D. Jakes
Woman, Thou Art Loosed

when they usually shrink even further secondary to the decreased levels of estrogen in the system.[5] It seems to me that starting progesterone in early perimenopause and keeping hormones balanced is a better choice than surgery. I believe in prevention.

Breast Pain and Fibrocystic Breast: The breast tissue is very sensitive to the stimulatory effects of estrogen.[6] Breasts can swell, enlarge, and become inflamed, tender, and painful when estrogen is dominant. Fibrocystic breast disease has been associated with a number of problems. Dr. Gary Null suggests in his book *Women's Health Solutions* that fibrocystic breast disease is caused by congestion from foods that clog the system such as wheat, dairy, refined foods, and fats. He also states that toxic accumulations called xenoestrogens (toxins that behave like estrogens) found in pesticides, fuels, and plastics can enhance the production of these so-called bad estrogens and bind to estrogen receptors, creating single or multiple breast lumps. These cysts/tumors are usually harmless but are associated with a higher than normal chance of developing into breast cancer at a later date.[7]

We have a lot of daily exposure to toxins (xenoestrogens) in our environment, in addition to the congesting foods mentioned by Dr. Null above. If one is already estrogen dominant during this particular time in one's life (perimenopause), then the combination of the two can definitely fuel the problem, especially when associated with high stress or the consumption of products such as caffeine, chocolate, and soft drinks. Although no hormone can make up for a poor diet, I believe that using bioidentical progesterone can certainly help oppose this estrogen dominance as well as the xenoestrogens in the system and give some protection.

Thyroid Dysfunction: Hypothyroidism is seven times more frequent among women than men, and I believe estrogen dominance influences thyroid dysfunction. Dr. Hotze says in *Hormones, Health, and Happiness:*

> When estrogen levels are high, the liver produces high levels of thyroid-binding globulin (TBG), the protein that binds to thyroid hormones in the blood and prevents them from being taken up by the cells. Women suffering from estrogen dominance may have a normally functioning thyroid gland

that produces adequate amounts of the thyroid hormones, and blood tests to measure levels of thyroid hormone and thyroid stimulating hormones may read as "normal." However, because the hormone is bound to and inactivated by the circulating proteins, little of it is actually getting into the cells.[8]

Further, estrogen and thyroid hormones compete for the same receptor sites. When there is too much estrogen in the system and the body is trying to balance out the hormones, secondary to the estrogen dominance, the receptor sites are *full* of estrogen, and there is nowhere for the thyroid hormone to go. There are not enough receptor sites to utilize the small amount of unbound, circulating thyroid hormone that is present. This exacerbates the situation even more, and a symptomatic hypothyroid condition can be present.[9] Balancing the hormones with bioidentical progesterone can reduce estrogen dominance and promote proper thyroid hormone uptake.

Osteoporosis: Again in *Hormones, Health, and Happiness,* Dr. Hotze states that conventional thinking in the medical community attributes osteoporosis to the decline in estrogen hormones that occurs in a woman's postmenopausal years. However, he believes this conventional thinking to be wrong. Women begin losing bone mineral density years before menopause, and Dr. Hotze believes that it is progesterone, not estrogen, that is the key to preventing osteoporosis. He states,

If estrogen were the most important hormone in maintaining bone health, then women would maintain their peak bone density until their fifties. They would experience bone loss only after menopause, when estrogen levels decline dramatically. However, this is not the case. … the decline in progesterone levels that occurs beginning in a woman's mid-thirties is a much more critical factor in causing bone loss than the decline in estrogen levels that occurs at menopause. This is due to the interaction of progesterone and estrogen with specialized bone cells called osteoclasts and osteoblasts. Ostesoclasts are responsible for breaking down old bone, while osteoblasts build new bone … Estrogen helps slow bone loss by curbing the activity of the bone-dissolving osteoclasts, but it has no effect on osteoblasts. On the other hand, progesterone attaches to specialized receptor sites on the surface of the osteoblasts and stimulates bone-building activity.[10]

Dr. Jane Guiltinan also notes in *Women's Health Solutions* by Dr. Null, "Estrogen minimizes calcium loss from bones, but progesterone can actually put calcium back into bones."[11] This is one of the primary reasons that I recommend women start supplementing with bioidentical progesterone at early perimenopause when progesterone levels start to decline. Although progesterone is only one piece of the bone-density puzzle, in terms of the role hormones play in the body for prevention of osteoporosis, I believe it to be a major piece.

Several other studies have demonstrated the stimulatory effects of both progesterone and estrogen in bone formation and mineralization. These studies have concluded that hormone replacement therapy decreases serum and urine markers of bone metabolism, prevents bone loss, and results in an increase in spine and hip bone mineral density.[12] Again, a good balance of both estrogen and progesterone, each playing their particular role at the correct stage, can help prevent this horrid disease we call osteoporosis.

Migraine Headaches: Migraine headaches can be another symptom of estrogen dominance. Too much estrogen can facilitate water retention, dilation of blood vessels, depletion of minerals such as magnesium, and constriction of the arteries. Dr. Hotze states,

> Estrogen promotes water retention. Because the brain is confined to the fixed space of the skull, when it swells the pressure that develops causes a headache. Estrogen also causes dilation of the blood vessels. The constriction of blood vessels followed by rebound dilation is a key factor in migraine headaches. Finally, estrogen dominance leads to depletion of the mineral magnesium, which is crucial to normal blood vessel tone. Magnesium deficiency can cause a spasm of arteries in the brain.[13]

The places we are seen and heard are holy places.
They remind us of our value as human beings. They
give us the strength to go on. Eventually they may
even help us transform our pain into wisdom.

—Rachel Naomi Remen, MD
Kitchen Table Wisdom
Stories That Heal

Further, Drs. Lee and Zava, in their book *What Your Doctor May Not Tell You About Breast Cancer,* articulate that women who suffer cyclical migraines that occur during the week or so just prior to their period will usually find relief by supplementing with progesterone during that time.[14] Again, balancing hormones with added progesterone and magnesium may keep migraines and menstrual headaches at bay during perimenopause as well as prior to menstrual periods in the childbearing years.

Low Libido: Estrogen dominance has a profound effect on one's libido by increasing levels of sex hormone-binding globulins. These are proteins that attach themselves to progesterone and testosterone and deactivate them. Now we all know that women are to a greater degree more emotional beings than men, so sexual desire for us does not entirely come from our sex hormones but from our brains. However, by eliminating estrogen dominance and progesterone deficiency, sexual desire can be improved.[15] Low libido is one of the most frequent complaints I hear in my practice. Most women with hormonal imbalances will admit they need all the help they can get in this department.

Bladder Health: Most of us over fifty years of age know that after menopause our bladder tone is not what it used to be. Many elderly women tend to be more susceptible to bladder infections. There is no magical answer for this because each woman's urinary tract and pelvic floor support is different. In my clinic, women who have had more children usually complain of stress incontinence and urine leakage slightly more (and earlier in life) than women who have not experienced childbirth. However, after hormones disappear, there is probably not much difference between the two according to what I observe on a regular basis.

Our female hormones are what help keep our bladder toned. In one Swedish study, with the use of vaginal estriol (a very mild form of estrogen), 75 percent of the women reported significant subjective improvement in stress incontinence.[16] In another study in Israel, it was concluded that vaginal estriol prevents the recurrence of urinary tract infections in postmenopausal women.[17] I have found this to be true among the women I treat in my clinic. BHRT (including combinations of estrogens and progesterone), estradiol, or estriol vaginal cream works well in helping to keep the bladder toned, reduce symptoms of what many women perceive to be a bladder infection, as well as reduce stress incontinence and urine leakage. Therefore, I think we may conclude that the use of bioidentical estrogen (balanced with progesterone) after menopause can benefit the urinary tract, in the form of both reducing stress incontinence and the overall health of the bladder. The risk of being embarrassed and not participating in certain activities secondary to this problem would definitely make one want to do everything possible to avoid this situation.

What about breast cancer risk?

Breast cancer is on the rise. Doesn't that tell you that we have a bigger problem out there than just hormones? "Estrogen alone does not cause breast cancer. If that were true, every 18-year-old would have cancer since that is the age when your estrogen levels are highest. Breast cancer is a complex process in which many factors combine to cause, what we know and call, cancer," says Dr. Edward J. Conley in his book *Safe Estrogen*.[18]

God, in His perfect design of the body (and I believe it was perfect before the fall), didn't give women hormones to cause cancers. Yes, an imbalance in hormones can promote tissue growth and growth of cancerous tumors, but hormones themselves do not *give* you cancer. Free radicals (negatively charged molecules that destroy DNA) cause cancer. We take trillions of free radical hits daily secondary to toxins from over-the-counter medications; prescribed medications; birth control pills; pollution of air, water, and foods; high-carbohydrate and sugary diets; pesticides; heavy metal exposure; plastics; and on and on we could go.

There is not one person out there who can completely isolate him or herself from the devastation of all of these toxins to which we are exposed. We would have to be living in an organic bubble of some sort. We can, however, do some things to support the body by getting rid of and oxidizing (inactivating) these free radicals to protect ourselves from the ravages of these toxins. I will talk about those things in a later chapter on toxicity, but let us get back to the main subject. Your own bioidentical hormones do not *cause* cancer. There has been a lot of misunderstanding out there on this subject, most likely because of the harmful effects of synthetics. Let us try and get away from that false information that *all* hormones are bad for you. As a matter of fact, the International Agency for Research on Cancer, which is part of the

The I in illness is isolation, and the
crucial letters in wellness are we.

—Author Unknown

World Health Organization (WHO), estimates that 25 to 30 percent of breast cancer cases could simply be avoided if women ate healthier and followed a regular exercise program.[19] So please, please, let us not blame cancer(s) on hormones as has been done in the past; it is just not true!

Cancer is caused by multiple factors. Hormones play a vital role in a person's overall general health, as we discussed earlier. Significant research has been done on synthetic hormones, and again, we know the outcome of the WHI study. Yes, synthetic hormones (which are medications that are chemically toxic to the system) can increase the risk of cancer. Taking *any* kind of toxic substance day-in and day-out, week after week, month after month, and year after year can create enough free radicals to start minute tumors in the body. But remember, I am talking about your own natural hormones and compounded hormones that are bioidentical in structure to what the body produces. If you choose to take hormones, it is important to choose BHRT. A provider that specializes in BHRT that is going to test and work with you continually to keep your hormones balanced properly is essential, even with BHRT.

Testing is a key component when it comes to hormones. Some clients who come to my clinic for the first time have been taking hormones for years without ever having had their levels checked, even on an occasional basis. Usually they are and have been having symptoms of hormone imbalance for years, whether it be weight gain, insomnia, hair growth/loss, fatigue, and so on, but no one has suggested that they actually check their hormone levels. Watching lab results is important for a good balance, in addition to monitoring clinical symptoms.

Estrogen Dominance: In my opinion, taking estrogen without balancing it with progesterone is harmful, even if you *do not* have a uterus. Think about it—if God made us to have a perfect *balance* of all hormones in the proper ratios during our childbearing years, then wouldn't it make sense (if we choose to take any kind of BHRT) that we need to balance *all* of the hormones (estrogen, progesterone, testosterone, etc.)? Dominance or deficiency in any of the hormones is not a good thing, regardless of whether a uterus is intact. However, if you do not check your hormone levels, then you will never know which hormones are deficient and where you need to supplement.

Clinically, I see that many women who are on estrogen-only supplementation have a very high estrone level, especially if they have been taking synthetic estrogens alone. Estrone is one of the three estrogens made by the body that is considered to be more cancer *promoting* (I didn't say producing). Even if you are taking BHRT, your levels need to be checked at least yearly, including your estrone levels, to determine if those levels are too high.

Additional Tests: Further, there are other clinical tests that can be taken to see how the body is metabolizing the hormones and whether the body is metabolizing them through the correct pathway. Each individual person's body has its own way of breaking down and metabolizing hormones depending on that person's overall health status. This is done in the liver. To simplify, estrogen is basically metabolized into two major pathways: the 16 OH (hydroxy) metabolite (the bad) and the 2 OH (hydroxy) metabolite (the good). Every woman converts some of the estrogen down each pathway, but you always want the good-to-bad ratio to be higher. Dr. Conley states,

> The 16 OH metabolite retains significant estrogen activity. In fact, some researchers feel it is actually more potent and more dangerous than estrogen itself! Studies have shown that overproduction of 16 OH significantly increases your risk of breast cancer. The 2 OH pathway, however, has been associated with a LOWER risk of breast cancer. Low levels of 2 OH have been associated with breast cancer, uterine cancer (also cervical cancer and lupus). Medical Studies have shown that the lower your 2 OH/16 OH ratio, especially if it is below 2, the HIGHER your risk of breast cancer.[20]

Checking the 2 OH/16 OH ratio is an indicator of how the body is metabolizing the estrogens, whether they are from endogenous (from the body) or exogenous (from outside the body) sources. If the ratio is off, it doesn't mean you have to stop taking your BHRT, but it would be a red flag that should make you wake up and take note of your personal health practices. Consider whether you are eating the correct type of diet and taking the right kinds of supplements needed to assist your body in operating properly for optimum health and wellness. There are a number of health-care practices that can dramatically change this ratio of metabolites for the better. I recommend that you spend the money to take a simple 2/16 OH ratio urine test even if you are not on BHRT, especially if your estrone levels are high. See appendix I for more information concerning this test and how to order.

As I stated earlier, breast cancer is not limited to women on hormone replacement therapy. Genetic predisposition plays a part, although this has been exaggerated, but environmental factors play the largest role in the development of all cancers, particularly breast cancer.[21] You do not want to be metabolizing those estrogens in a pathway that would increase or speed up the growth of any minute tumors present. You want to do everything you can to balance and prevent.

Hysterectomies: Many practitioners treat their hysterectomized patients with estradiol only. The rationale for this is that if a woman does not have a uterus to protect, the progesterone or progestin component is unnecessary. But what about the breasts, as well as the brain, lungs, and other parts of the body that have estrogen receptors? Those sites need to be protected too! We've already established above that estrogen dominance is detrimental to a woman's body and puts one at a higher risk for promoting cancer growth. The proper balance between estrogen and progesterone (the hormone that opposes estrogen) is an important component.

Again, testing is the key. If a good balance of hormones plays an important role in your overall general health and wellness and you have chosen BHRT, tests must be performed at least yearly. This assures that both the estrogen and progesterone and any other hormone(s) that you may be using are in balance and stay in balance and that their dominance of one or the other is kept in check. Again, in *What Your Doctor May Not Tell You about Breast Cancer,* the authors state,

A rational approach to hormone therapy would include tests of free hormone levels so that hormone supplements are used only for women truly hormone deficient, and in doses that restore normal physiologic levels, rather than the "one-dose-fits-all" approach. Conventional medicine projects a dilemma: how to supplement estrogen without increasing estrogen-induced risk. The dilemma may be a mirage created by overdosing. With proper endogenous hormone balance during the premenopause years, women remain healthy. Why wouldn't the same be true if proper hormone balance is achieved during postmenopausal years?[22]

Further, studies have shown that hormone replacement therapy (HRT) use in women with a family history of breast cancer is not associated with any significant increase in breast cancer but is actually associated with a significantly reduced mortality rate.[23] Adding progestogens may even decrease the recurrence of breast cancer.[24] Dr. Conley notes a study published by the American Journal of Epidemiology showed women who were deficient in progesterone are five times more likely to get breast cancer than women who were not deficient.[25] Dr. John R. Lee wrote in one of his most recent blogs that he finds the saliva progesterone level in healthy women to be two hundred to three hundred times greater than the saliva estradiol levels. In women with breast cancer, that ratio is considerably less than two hundred to one.[26] Again, bioidentical progesterone can give some protection to the breasts (as well as other organs) by alleviating the progesterone deficiency and correcting the estrogen dominance.

In conclusion, balance on all levels is the key. Hormones in the body should be kept or restored to their normal physiologic levels. If this is the goal that you and your provider are working to achieve, hormones will not be a contributing factor to breast cancer or any other cancer. Having a professional health-care provider who is knowledgeable in BHRT, hormone testing, and the clinical signs and symptoms of hormone imbalance and who is truly working for your benefit is essential for your overall health and decision making when it comes to BHRT.

Will BHRT help your memory?

Personally speaking, I could not remember how to get out of bed in the morning if I had to give up my bioidentical hormones. I understand that keeping my hormones correctly balanced affords me more energy and a better outlook on life; and additionally, my memory is considerably better! It is widely known that our hormones peak in our twenties and begin to slowly decline thereafter. This decline in youthful peaks can bring on symptoms such as lower energy levels, weight gain, moodiness, difficulty thinking and concentrating, and poor memory.[27] When you

Exercise daily,
walk with the Lord.

—Author Unknown

enter menopause where there is not just a decline in hormones but when production of hormones from the ovaries have disappeared altogether, it can get even worse.

One clinical study has concluded,

> Estrogen specifically maintains verbal memory
> in women and may prevent or forestall the
> deterioration in short- and long-term memory
> that occurs with normal aging. There is also
> evidence that estrogen decreases the incidence
> of Alzheimer disease or retards its onset or
> both.[28]

I have read additional studies that showed that too much estrogen or estrogen dominance actually has the opposite effect. So once again, I infer that when you consider brain function, you need to consider balance of both progesterone and estrogen according to testing and clinical symptoms.

What about taking birth control pills (BCPs) for perimenopausal symptoms?

Again, BCPs are synthetic hormones, and as you can already guess, I am certainly against that. If you are trying to improve your health and not destroy it or place as few toxins in the body as you have control over, then BCPs would be on the top of the list of "What Not to Take!" However, on the facts-of-the-matter level, perimenopause is a time of uncertain ovulation, with lower progesterone levels and estrogen dominance. Many women are concerned about pregnancy during the premenopausal years. Progesterone therapy is the hormone of choice during this particular time for symptoms and balance, although it is not sufficient for birth control. Even with my younger clients who feel that BCPs are their best option for family planning, I have always maintained that BCPs should be viewed as short-term therapy, limited to one to three years use. Five is stretching it in my opinion. Perimenopause can last for ten to fifteen years, depending on the individual. The symptoms of perimenopause can begin in the mid to late thirties and last until menopause, which could be at fifty-two years old on average or twelve to fifteen years. That is a long time to be taking BCPs (synthetic hormones), thus increasing your chances of cancers, not to mention all of the symptoms and negative side effects that I see many women experiencing that go along with synthetic hormone use, such as low libido, depression, and moodiness.

Dr. Pamela Smith states in her book, *HRT: The Answer* that BCPs containing estrogen decrease vitamins B12, folate, and B6 in your body, which are needed to metabolize homocysteine. If homoscysteine builds up in your system, it can predispose you to heart disease and Alzheimer's. BCPs also deplete the body of zinc, increase copper levels, and decrease serum testosterone and dehydroepiandrosterone (DHEA). Dr. Smith further states that BCPs contain synthetic progestins, which decrease the positive effects of estrogen on your heart, and that even low-dose BCPs contain more estrogens and progestin than is usually needed for treatment of perimenopause or menopause.[29]

Please also remember that perimenopause is a time to be thinking about the positive things you can do for your health. I always remind my clients that the lifestyle changes that are made for the better during this time will greatly affect their quality of life postmenopause and beyond. However, if you do choose or have chosen to take BCPs during perimenopause, please make sure it is for a very brief time until you can search out a holistic health care provider who will help get you on the right track with the bioidentical hormone options and counsel you on alternative birth control methods, preferably ones free from synthetic hormones.

What about taking herbs or soy?

Many women have asked me over the years about taking herbal or soy products for menopausal symptoms. I really have no big problem with these products, but I believe that women should use them with caution. There are a number of herbal and soy products that either by themselves or in combination with other herbs, vitamins, and minerals can help to calm symptoms and balance hormones a bit. These products usually take several months of use (at least three months) to achieve a significant therapeutic level to do the job. Women who experience more severe symptoms than average may find these products are not effective enough to make them as comfortable and symptom-free as they want

For attractive lips, speak words of kindness.

For lovely eyes, seek out the good in people.

For a slim figure, share your food with the hungry.

For beautiful hair, let a child run his/her fingers
through it once a day.

For poise, walk with the knowledge that you never
walk alone.

People, even more than things, have to be restored,
renewed, revived, reclaimed, and redeemed; never
throw out anyone.

As you grow older, you will discover that you have
two hands, one for helping yourself; and one for
helping others.

—Audrey Hepburn

to be. Some herbal products indicated for menopausal symptoms would include, but are not limited to, soy and herbs such as don quai, black cohosh, ginseng, alfalfa, black haw, fennel, red clover, and licorice.[30] If you use a pure product, as I discuss in chapter 9, then you may find these products very helpful for the relief of mild to moderate symptoms. Please be advised that some herbal products contain blood-thinning properties, so they should be stopped at least two weeks prior to any medical procedure or surgery.

There is no over-the-counter herb supplement that actually contains estrogen. However, the herbs listed above contain phytoestrogens that mimic or interact with estrogen hormones. There are about three hundred plants that have been identified to contain these compounds. When eaten or taken in as part of a normal diet, phytoestrogens are safe and beneficial. They are easily broken down, are not stored in tissue, and spend very little time in the body. However, when phytoestrogens are taken in large doses for menopausal symptoms, such as those found in herbal capsules, they behave like estrogens in the body and alter hormone-dependent tissue function.[31] These larger doses can definitely give some symptom relief but may also create enough estrogenic action to stimulate the uterus and thicken the uterine lining. That is why these herbs are contraindicated in women who have endometriosis. Without balancing this herbal intake with progesterone to keep the uterine lining thin, one may possibly be increasing one's chances for uterine cancer. If I have a client who tells me she is on an herbal product known to have even weak estrogenic action, I highly recommend that she balance the product with some bioidentical progesterone.

Although soy is not an herb, soy contains very high levels of phytoestrogens.[32] If I have a client who has a significant daily intake of soy (other than what is in a normal diet, as discussed above), I recommend that she take progesterone. I have talked about the effect on the uterus, but these herb and soy phytoestrogens can also stimulate breast tissue and may cause breast tenderness. I hate to keep repeating myself, but again, balance is the key. Even with herbs and soy, you do not want to take any chances of doing anything that would throw off that delicate balance and create problems later. Taking these products alone would cause the same effects as an estrogen-dominant situation, as discussed earlier.

Also remember that wild yam is not a natural source of progesterone. Although a pharmaceutical process can produce bioidentical progesterone from wild yams, the body cannot duplicate this conversion.[33] So when you are looking to use natural progesterone to balance your estrogenic herbs or soy, it must be a bioidentical United States Pharmaceutical Grade (USP) micronized progesterone source and not a wild yam cream. Although lower doses of USP micronized progesterone can be bought over the counter, my recommendation is that you should always work with a provider who uses a certified compounding pharmacy. He or she can assess your particular situation and make sure you are getting the correct products, amount, and balance of both herbs and progesterone.

What is the bottom line on hormones?

Your body needs bioidentical hormones for optimal health and wellness. I believe from my research and clinical experience that keeping your hormones in balance will help in this process. In order to do so, you must work with someone who is experienced in the field of hormone and whole-system balancing, who will order the necessary testing, and who will work with you to correct the particular imbalances that may exist in the body. I have a firm conviction that just balancing hormones is only a part of the events that need to take place to achieve the health status we all desire. Working on other systems (as I pray you learn about in this book) is absolutely as necessary as balancing your hormones. When whole-system balancing is the utmost priority, the synergy of the hormones, nutrition, and supplements will create a symphony of the body's systems that can be amazing!

God would prefer we have an occasional limp than a perpetual strut. And if it takes a thorn for Him to make His point, He loves us enough not to pluck it out.

—Max Lucado
Let the Journey Begin

Chapter 2

❧

Heart Health and Beyond

Heart disease is the number-one killer among both men and postmenopausal women and the leading cause for disability. About every twenty-five seconds, an American will have a heart attack, and about one will die every minute.[1] I probably do not have to tell you the underlying cause of this problem: to the greater extent, the American diet. With all the technology, drugs, and treatments that the traditional medical community has in its possession, the risk of heart disease is not necessarily getting better. Although death rates from coronary artery disease and stroke decreased slightly in 2010 (still the number-one killer), they did not reach the benchmark for which researchers had hoped. As a matter of fact, the United States performed so poorly in other areas of women's health, such as obesity, hypertension, diabetes, and binge drinking, that even though there was that slight improvement in deaths from heart disease in 2010, it is expected those numbers will go right back up in 2011.[2]

Although many of us try to watch our diets and eat healthy, the American diet has changed dramatically over the past fifty years. It is a commonly known fact that our foods contain much less nutritional value than they did twenty or thirty years ago. Obesity in children is rampant, and now we have a new generation with a whole set of new disease processes directly related to the lack of nutrition in the American diet. For instance, fifty years ago diabetes was a disease that one was either born with (type I diabetes) or maybe eventually developed in old age (type II diabetes). Now we are seeing a trend where children and young adults are developing insulin resistance and diabetes in their early teens and twenties, which is believed to be directly related to diet and nutrition. It is not just children; the adult population in America is obese too, and that is causing many health problems.

Yes, we are the richest and most well fed but unfortunately also one of the fattest nations on earth, with 74.1 percent of those over fifteen years old considered to be overweight![3] I do believe that genetics play a part in whether a person is obese or develops a particular disease, but I also firmly believe we give genetics way too much credit over our environmental factors these days, and unfortunately, we sometimes use them as an excuse for a poor diet and not enough exercise. Until we can reverse those lifestyle trends and work on prevention measures, I believe heart disease will continue to rise.

I recognize that there are a number of variables that are to blame in the development of heart disease. However, I would like to cover a few key topics that I believe play a more significant role in the development of heart disease in the postmenopausal woman and how low hormones, nutrient deficiencies, and dietary excess may relate to these conditions.

Major Risk Factors

Insulin Resistance/Type II Diabetes: Insulin resistance is a term used when the number of insulin receptors on your cells decrease. Without enough insulin receptor sites on each cell's surface, glucose cannot properly be utilized by the body. Glucose then remains in the blood stream, often causing elevated blood sugar levels. The body has to do something with the extra glucose, so it is sent to the liver, where it is converted to fat and stored throughout the body. In *Women's Bodies, Women's Wisdom*, Dr. Christiane Northrup states,

> Chief among the risk factors for heart disease is increased insulin resistance, which is present to some degree in 50 to 75 percent of women in this country. The problem with high insulin (which is initially protective) and over consumption of carbohydrates result in increased body fat and aberrations in lipid profile.[4]

In other words, too much insulin causes levels of triglycerides and the low-density lipoproteins (LDLs)—the bad cholesterol—to go up and your levels of high-density lipoproteins (HDLs)—the good cholesterol—to go down. Some additional effects caused by too much insulin can be sodium retention, which may promote high blood pressure, an increase in uric acid, and gouty arthritis, and an increased inflammatory response throughout the body and arteries, which can lead to heart disease. Not only does insulin resistance play a role in the aforementioned, it can also lead to abdominal obesity and the increased risk of developing type II diabetes and stroke. The combination of these symptoms is frequently referred to as syndrome X,[5] and more recently metabolic syndrome or insulin resistance.

Having your fasting insulin and hemoglobin A1C levels checked yearly is a good way to find out if you are at risk. If your levels are borderline high, then you have an opportunity to correct the problem before it is too late. That is what preventative medicine is all about—knowing where the problems lie and then doing something about them before they get out of control. Getting your insulin and blood sugars under control at this point is relatively easy with the right diet and exercise program. There are also a number of nutritional supplements that further support the utilization of sugar and insulin in the body. A good holistic health-care practitioner can help you decide what supplements would best suit you.

I have read a number of articles that present information that *too high* estrogens or androgens in the system may contribute to insulin resistance. Again, the words *too high* indicate an imbalance in hormones. There is increasing evidence linking endogenous estrogen 17B-estradiol to the maintenance and homeostasis (a stable state of equilibrium) of glucose. Postmenopausal women have a tendency toward visceral obesity and insulin resistance and are at risk for type II diabetes, but hormone replacement therapy leads to a reduction in the incidence of diabetes. This particular study has shed light on the anti-diabetic properties of estradiol at tissue-specific levels.[6] In other words, hormones balanced and in the right proportions actually help to stabilize and maintain proper glucose levels.

When it comes to eating right and exercising, there is no "I'll start tomorrow." Tomorrow is disease.

—Terri Guillemets

Cholesterol: Is it good or is it bad? That is the question that can be so confusing at times for perimenopause and post-menopausal women. Cholesterol levels frequently tend to rise in a number of women as they begin to approach menopause. Cholesterol itself is really a good thing. But as I always say, "Too much of a good thing can sometimes be, well, too much." However, in late perimenopause and early postmenopause, higher cholesterol levels *are* a good thing. Listen to me—I said higher, not exceptionally high.

In God's great design of our magnificent human body, cholesterol plays a very important role in the manufacturing of hormones in the adrenal system. I mention in a later chapter on the adrenals that all the adrenal hormones start with cholesterol. Without going into all of the physiology of how cholesterol is made and all of its many other important functions in the body, I want to concentrate on how cholesterol affects us at perimenopause and postmenopause. Cholesterol is an important precursor for the synthesis of steroid hormones, including the adrenal gland hormones cortisol and aldosterone, as well as the sex hormones progesterone, estradiol, testosterone, and their derivatives.[7]

Chapter 1 also reviews that once the ovaries cease to make the necessary hormones to carry out the biochemical processes needed for optimum health, the adrenals have to take over that job. Besides doing all of the normal functions that the adrenals have been doing all of your life, they now have the additional burden of producing the sex hormones. Consequently, cholesterol is *the* much-needed precursor because suddenly the body needs these hormones to function correctly. The body's survival mechanisms kick in and start producing more cholesterol so that the adrenals can take on this extra task. Cholesterol levels rise and come to the rescue. In this case, *higher* cholesterol levels are good and present the natural and expected bodily response to the now lower hormone levels.

I have noticed that initiation of BHRT causes cholesterol levels to return to more normal levels, although they are slightly higher than prior to menopause. The reason for this is that most health-care providers (such as myself) who initiate BHRT are not trying to restore hormone levels back to what they were in the childbearing years. The therapy goal should be mild to moderate dosings that create therapeutic levels to calm symptoms, support the adrenals, and thus help the body function more optimally—but again, not at the levels that were present in our twenties and thirties needed for fertility purposes. At this time in a woman's life, slightly higher levels of cholesterol are to be expected and are purposeful to produce additional hormones on days when our hormone levels that are being taking exogenously may fall short secondary to stress, poor nutrition, poor absorption, or other life factors.

Traditional medical providers often fail to take this into account for late-perimenopausal and postmenopausal women and many times suggest a cholesterol-lowering medication. If that is the case, the much-needed extra cholesterol plummets as a result of the medication and sends the system into further distress. Without enough cholesterol, there will be fewer steroid and sex hormones made that promote optimum health and a properly functioning system. The bottom line on the subject of cholesterol is that you must take into account where you are in this life span of hormones when looking at total cholesterol numbers as well as the HDLs and LDLs. It is estimated that 50 percent of those who suffer heart attacks have normal cholesterol numbers and that 30 percent of the population has cholesterol-depleted LDLs (a condition where the cholesterol may be normal, but the lipoprotein particle number is much higher, thus an unexpected elevated risk of cardiovascular disease). Advanced testing can now be done on these smaller lipoprotein particles to assess these risks. It is these lipoprotein particles that are responsible for key steps in plaque formation and the resulting development of heart disease. Measuring these lipoprotein subgroups is the best way to evaluate new risk factors and really determine if a cholesterol-lowering medication will be of more benefit than nutritional and/or lifestyle changes.[8]

In my opinion, if it is not genetic or if you really need to lower your cholesterol levels considerably and are also serious about making the necessary changes, the majority of the time it can be done the natural way without introducing drugs and subsequent toxins in your system. Balancing hormones, improving diet, adding the appropriate supplementation, and exercising are great places to start. If it is determined that you must take cholesterol-lowering medication(s), whether for familial hyperlipidemia or secondary to hormonal changes in the body, hopefully it will only be short term until the levels can be brought under control with more natural means. And since cholesterol

Half the modern drugs could be thrown out the window, except that the birds might eat them.

—Martin H. Fisher

drugs have side effects and are very toxic to the liver, it is important to remember to detoxify the liver twice yearly. Also take a nano-CoQ10 because this nutrient is depleted by cholesterol-lowering drugs. Again, a holistic health-care provider can help you determine the best way(s) to accomplish this task.

Stress: What exactly is stress? Like cholesterol, is it good or bad? I know that stress is a frequently used word. We hear, "I'm all stressed out," on a daily basis. We have our good days and our not-so-good days. We all know that life happens! But do the not-so-good days constitute stress? When we experience stress, whether from a physical or emotional standpoint, the body goes into the fight-or-flight response. This is a natural response to handle the present situation by releasing the major stress hormones adrenaline and cortisol, as well as others called eicosanoids.[9] This fight-or-flight response is certainly good for that particular situation and for a short period of time, but long term it is detrimental to your health and considered to be one of the major risk factors for heart disease. Adrenaline is released from the body quickly, but cortisol sticks around for a while. Dr. Hotze states,

> Adrenaline's effects are dramatic and unmistakable, but because this hormone does not linger in your body, its effects are also relatively short-lived. On the other hand, cortisol, the stress hormone produced by the outer cortex, has more prolonged effects on your body. If adrenaline is like that whip that drives the horse faster and faster, cortisol is like the rider's boot, digging into the flank, keeping the horse going even when it's ready to quit.[10]

He further adds that chronically elevated levels of cortisol can be extremely damaging due to its metabolic effects. People with this problem may develop high blood sugar and insulin levels, may gain weight around the waistline, and have a greater risk of heart disease.[11] Most likely you have seen people in this constant state of stress and commented that if they didn't de-stress or slow down, they were going to have a heart attack. That *is* true; chronic stress can lead to abnormal blood clotting factors and plaqueing of the arteries, which can lead to heart disease.[12] Keeping hormones balanced is a good way to decrease stress in one's life. Women who keep their hormones in balance are less likely to have the symptoms that cause a lot of emotional as well as physical stress, such as fatigue, depression, moodiness, anxiety, and weight gain.

As we can all agree, there are times when we do not have control over a number of our stressors. However, we do have a God who is *in control* and much bigger than our problems. Daily meditating on and being in His Word can greatly help us give over and release to Him some of these situations we face daily. Christ said in Matthew 6:25–27, "Therefore I tell you, do not worry about your life … who of you by worrying can add a single hour to his life?" (NIV). And Matthew 11:28–30 says, "Come unto me all you who are weary and burdened and I will give you rest. Take my yoke upon you and learn from me for I am gentle and humble in heart and you will find rest for your souls. For my yoke is easy and my burden is light" (NIV). This releasing-to-God thing definitely needs practice. But we can do it! In this day and age, we so desperately need that rest for our bodies *and* our souls. If we make it a habit to start our day with praise to the Father for His provision and the awareness that there is divine control in our lives, we are less likely to practice the bad habit of stressing out.

High Blood Pressure/Hypertension: It is a fact that people with higher blood pressure have higher rates of heart disease and stroke. When we take our blood pressure, we get a two-number reading, such as 120/80. The top number is the systolic pressure number, and the bottom number is the diastolic pressure. Anything equal to or greater than 140 systolic pressure and anything equal to or greater than 90 diastolic is considered high blood pressure or hypertension. Clinically, these high readings must be observed on at least three occasions to establish the diagnosis of hypertension.[13] The systolic pressure is the pressure that is exerted against the arteries when the heart squeezes the blood from the heart. The diastolic number is the pressure against the arteries when the heart is at rest or is between beats. Blood pressure readings are dependent on the strength of the heartbeat, the elasticity or flexibility of the walls of the arteries, and the amount and thickness of the blood flowing through the vessels.[14]

There are arguments about which number is the most important—that is, whether systolic or diastolic pressure is more meaningful or what some now call the pulse pressure. Pulse pressure is the number you get when you subtract the diastolic pressure number from the systolic pressure number.[15] I am not here to argue one point or the other; however, it sure makes a lot of common sense that if a high pressure is being exerted on the vessels at any point and in any case, more damage will be done to the walls of the arteries. It is these damaged vessel areas where plaqueing begins and thus atherosclerosis.

Like many other diseases, hypertension and heart disease do not begin overnight. It develops over a long period of time secondary to "dietary habits, lack of exercise, high stress, being overweight, having too much caffeine, sugar, alcohol, … [and] salt in the diet," says Dr. Gary Null.[16] Wow, after reading that list, it seems as if we are all doomed. But with God's help in a disciplined life, we can avoid this dreaded disease by changing some of the things we *can* control.

Research or sound written proof that hormones help with hypertension is lacking. There are some studies out there, however, that suggest potential advantages of blood pressure control by using natural progesterone.[17] I have experienced this to be true in the clinical setting. A number of patients whose blood pressures rose at late perimenopause or the beginning of menopause experienced normalized pressures once their hormones were balanced. Again, I think hormones in women are too often overlooked when such situations arise, especially in women who never experienced these problems prior to the drastic hormonal changes associated with late perimenopause and menopause. If this is you, and depending on your circumstances, it certainly may be helpful to balance your hormones, adjust your dietary habits, and see what happens before choosing a drug for correction. If your pressures are extremely high, hopefully medication will be a short-term solution while other things, such as hormones and lifestyle habits, are being brought under control. Remember to never stop your blood pressure medications abruptly. These medications must be weaned down under the supervision of a medical provider.

The. . .patient should be made to understand that he or she must take charge of his own life. Don't take your body to the doctor as if he were a repair shop.

—Quentin Regestein

Secondary Risk Factors

Homocysteine: Homocysteine is an amino acid produced by ineffective protein metabolism that promotes free radical production. Free radicals are negatively charged molecules that circulate throughout the body causing damage to the cell DNA, which can lead to a number of cancers and degenerative diseases, such as hardening of the arteries, heart disease, Alzheimer's, arthritis, and other inflammatory processes. These molecules are unstable and highly reactive and cause oxidation in our tissues. Oxidation is the same process that causes metals to rust and oil to become rancid. This process happening in our body secondary to this free radical damage can have devastating effects on our tissues and organs.[18]

According to Dr. Pamela Smith in her book *HRT: The Answers*, studies suggest that 42 percent of strokes, 28 percent of peripheral vascular disease, and approximately 30 percent of cardiovascular disease are directly related to elevated homocysteine levels.[19] Homocysteine tends to increase with menopause as well as for other reasons, such as hypothyroidism, during the use of certain prescribed drugs, exposure to environmental toxins, smoking, and kidney failure. There seems to be some genetic predisposition too. Before menopause, homocysteine levels tend to be lower. However, as estrogen levels drop, homocysteine levels tend to rise. Conversely, any situation that decreases estrogen or elevates testosterone levels can increase homocysteine in both pre- and postmenopausal women. Studies have shown that taking hormone replacement therapy lowers homocysteine levels.[20] Adequate intake of B vitamins such as B-6, B-12, and folic acid is essential for the breakdown of homocysteine in the body as well.[21] To repeat, balanced hormones, proper nutrition, and supplementation are needed to ensure normal homocysteine levels.

C-Reactive Protein: Research scientists believe that inflammation can cause heart disease. Recent research links high blood levels of C-reactive protein to heart attacks and stroke. Inflammation of the coronary arteries influences the buildup of arterial plaque and whether unstable patches of plaque are likely to break away, which can trigger a heart attack or stroke.[22] Inflammation is a complex biological response of tissue to harmful stimuli. Acute inflammation can be a good thing if you are trying to heal a wound. However, unchecked chronic inflammation in the body can cause a host of diseases, one being atherosclerosis, as well as heart valve dysfunction, obesity, and chronic heart failure.[23]

Some common causes of chronic inflammation in the body are chlamydia and herpes (sexually transmitted diseases), cytomegalovirus (a viral genus of the herpes family), chronic gum disease, and *Helicobacter pylori* (a bacteria responsible for chronic stomach inflammation) infection in the intestines. Also, oxidative as well as emotional stress can cause free radical damage and play a part in inflammation. C-reactive protein is an antibody-like substance that detects the presence of infection in the body. Higher levels of C-reactive protein reflect inflammation in the body and thus a higher risk for heart disease.[24]

The article "Effects of Transdermal Estradiol and Oral Conjugated Estradiol on C-reactive protein in Retinoid-Placebo Trial in Healthy Women" concluded that after twelve months of transdermal estradiol (bioidentical estrogen) therapy, there was no elevation of C-reactive protein. However, the oral conjugated equine estrogen (synthetic estrogen) did raise C-reactive protein levels by 48 percent in six months and 64 percent in twelve months, relative to a baseline.[25]

Therefore, if you choose hormone replacement therapy, stick with bioidentical estrogen (balanced with progesterone) because we know that synthetics increase inflammation in the system. Taking bioidentical estradiol does not raise C-reactive protein. Further, antioxidant supplementation can help reduce oxidative stress and free radical damage. As well, adhere to a diet *free* of polyunsaturated vegetable oils and trans-fatty acids, which are known to promote inflammation.

Fibrinogen: Fibrinogen is a clot-promoting substance in the blood. For women, this factor is worrisome because the more viscous (thicker) the blood, the easier clots can form and the higher the possibility of a stroke or heart attack. We have been led to believe that clotting is higher in women on hormone replacement therapy, and that is true if you are using the synthetic forms of hormones. The WHI study previously discussed used conjugated equine estrogen (made from pregnant horse mare urine) and/or medroxyprogesterone acetate, both synthetic hormones. The WHI Data and Safety Board stopped one arm of the study in 2002 because of the increased risks of blood clots as well as heart attacks and strokes.[26]

According to Dr. Pamela Smith, fibrinogen increases when estrogen levels decrease and fibrinogen decreases with bioidentical estrogen replacement therapy.[27] There are other nutritional factors that affect this too. The point is, BHRT can help with clotting factors. It is that balance game we must play again. If you have *too much* estrogen or estrogen dominance, most likely clotting factors will increase (thicker blood). Likewise, if you have *too little,* as Dr. Smith explained above, clotting factors will rise (thicker blood). I concur that you need a nice balance, as has been encouraged again and again in this book, to keep the blood less viscous and flowing smoothly. I also realize that there are many other factors that increase blood thickness, such as certain pathogens like fungi, viruses, parasites, and bacteria, certain ethnicities, certain genetic disorders, and heavy metal toxicity.[28] However, in terms of female hormones, I hope to convince you of the benefits that they provide your body in general and suggest that blame not be placed on natural hormones for all the ills women could possibly face, as some would like to do.

Excess Iron: Recent studies have shown that too much iron can increase the risk of heart disease. Every 1 percent increase (above normal levels) in ferritin can cause a 4 percent increase in the risk of a heart attack. When women stop menstruation, they have no reason to take iron supplements unless blood tests show they are iron deficient and they have been instructed to do so by their doctor.[29] This is why I discourage my postmenopausal clients from taking iron supplements or multi-vitamins that contain iron. If testing reveals that iron stores are deficient, I place them on iron therapy until further tests determine that levels have normalized. Then the supplementation is stopped.

Many women I speak with are confused on this subject. Most think that taking iron is healthy and often do so in their multi-vitamins or with additional supplementation. When women are young and still menstruating, a little iron probably does no harm. After menopause arrives and menstruation ceases, anemia is less likely and women may not need additional iron.[30] It is only suitable to take iron supplements if levels are low, whether menstruating or not.

As I have previously explained, many perimenopausal women tend to experience heavier bleeding issues secondary to estrogen dominance and the low progesterone levels. This certainly can cause a reduction in

Diseases of the soul are more dangerous and more numerous than those of the body.

—Cicero

iron stores, and adding an iron supplement short-term, when needed is warranted. However, Dr. Duane Graveline believes that an escalation of cardiovascular risk in postmenopausal women follows significant stored iron after menses cessation. He further states that this risk may be due to the inflammatory effects of stored iron and not cholesterol, as previously believed.[31] I recommend measuring serum ferritin, which (other than a bone marrow examination) is the most valuable indicator of iron stores in the body.[32] From this test, your provider will know whether supplementation is appropriate. If you are in perimenopause with excessive bleeding, adding progesterone may help balance hormones, reduce the flow, and prevent an anemic condition from occurring.

Some women beyond early menopause may become anemic with low iron levels secondary to a decrease in intrinsic factor in the gut. Intrinsic factor decreases vitamin B-12 absorption, thus causing pernicious anemia and the need for iron supplementation. It is unknown whether balancing hormones would rid the body of this potential. Again, your health-care provider can distinguish the problem with lab tests and direct you to the correct supplementation accordingly.

Conclusion

Women can reduce their chances of getting heart disease by taking the necessary steps mentioned above to prevent and control certain factors that put them at greater risk. Further, balancing hormones has positive heart health benefits. There are many studies that demonstrate the cardiovascular effects of hormones. It is no secret that menopausal women have a higher incidence of cardiovascular disease, and that is concerning; however, bioidentical hormone replacement therapy has actually been shown to have cardio-*protective* effects.[33] I realize that the hormone debate will continue to go on and on unnecessarily. But more and more physiological data and clinical outcomes demonstrate that bioidentical hormones are associated with lower risks of cardiovascular disease (as well as breast cancer) and are more efficacious than their synthetically derived counterparts.[34] In chapter 1, I discussed a number of other benefits of taking BHRT, but the cardio-*protective* effects are another reason, I believe, that supports the balancing of hormones when needed both before, at, and after menopause.

Man is born broken. He lives by mending.
The grace of God is glue.

—Eugene O'Neill
What's So Amazing about Grace?

Chapter 3

&

Hypothyroidism

Thyroid function is one of the most important functions in the body. It drives every biochemical process needed for life and optimum health. Maintaining balanced thyroid hormone levels is essential for this. It is estimated that in the general population, 10 percent of Americans have a low thyroid condition. This considers only those Americans who have actually been *diagnosed* with a hypothyroid condition and are on medication.[1] It has been my experience that many other Americans, and especially women, are *undiagnosed* secondary to many providers relying only on the blood test that measures TSH (thyroid stimulating hormone), while ignoring other signs and symptoms and more reliable tests that may lead to a better assessment of an underactive thyroid. In that case, this may mean that there are millions of adults (and possibly some children) out there who have an *undiagnosed* hypothyroid condition.

Other providers agree with this consensus. Dr. Brownstein states in *Overcoming Thyroid Conditions* that the true figure for hypothyroidism in America is closer to 40 percent of the population or approximately 52 million adults.[2] I have read other articles that believe this number to be even higher. If this is such a prevalent condition and many Americans are walking around *undiagnosed*, how can you make sure that you are not one of them? Let me explain in further detail how the thyroid works and answer some of those questions for you.

What does the thyroid gland do, and why do you need thyroid hormones?

The butterfly-shaped thyroid gland sits at the base of the neck and produces the thyroid hormones. The two major hormones are thyroxin (T4) and triiodothyronine (T3). Thyroid hormones work in every cell in the body (muscles, organs, heart, brain, and bones) and drive the metabolism in these cells. Without thyroid hormones or an adequate amount of thyroid hormones, metabolism becomes very sluggish and the body does not function optimally.

The thyroid gland makes approximately 80 percent of T4 and 20 percent T3. However, T3 is the more active form of the thyroid hormones that actually increases metabolism inside the cells. T4 is converted by the body to T3. There are other factors that I will discuss later in the chapter that affect this conversion, but in short, the conversion from T4 to T3 is made possible by an enzyme called 5'-deodinase (5'D-I) that is found in the organs of the body, such as the kidneys, liver, heart, and brain. In this process iodine is removed from T4, producing T3. If this enzyme malfunctions (regardless the reason), then less of the T4 is converted to T3. Since T3 is the most active form of the thyroid hormones and is the hormone that is taken up at the cellular level to carry out all of the metabolic functions, then there will be lower levels of or virtually no T3. At this point, a hypothyroid condition exists even if the TSH levels are within normal range.[3]

How does the thyroid-stimulating hormone (TSH) work?

TSH is secreted from a tiny gland in the center of the brain called the pituitary. The pituitary is very sensitive to changes in the levels of thyroid hormones in the body, and by stepping up or slowing down the production of TSH, it can regulate thyroid hormone production. If the pituitary gland is diseased or fails to produce the necessary TSH, the thyroid gland has no way of knowing that it needs to produce thyroid hormones and will not produce the needed hormones, even if blood levels drop.[4] This situation is considered a brain problem and must be dealt with immediately. However, assuming that the pituitary gland is functioning properly, it will signal the thyroid gland to perform its duties accordingly. TSH works on an inverse relationship. It will rise (the TSH level will increase) when the pituitary senses that the body needs to produce more thyroid hormone, and it will go down (the TSH level will decrease) if the pituitary senses it has enough or too much of the thyroid hormones. Many conventional medical providers use the TSH as their "gold standard" for assessing thyroid function. However, using the TSH only and ignoring other important tests, factors, and symptoms, I believe, results in many *under* and *undiagnosed* cases of hypothyroidism in many women (and men). Other tests in combination with the TSH, such as free T3, free T4, thyroid antibodies, and reverse T3, as well as clinical symptoms, can better assess thyroid function.

The typical reference range for TSH at this time is approximately .45 to 4.5ng/dl. This reference range can vary slightly from lab to lab. When you consider that the thyroid gland only produces a teaspoon of thyroid hormones in a year, then you can see why a small change in thyroid levels can have a significant effect on your body's metabolic function and ultimately your overall general health. Dr. Brownstein writes,

The thyroid gland secretes approximately one teaspoon of thyroid hormones over an entire year. This teaspoon of thyroid hormones must drive the metabolic rate of every cell in the body. Small variations in this amount will have wide ramifications on the health of the individual. It is impossible for the body to function at an optimum level of health if there is inadequate production of thyroid hormone.[5]

Let me offer you an example of the misuse of TSH testing. For instance, if your TSH at the age of forty is 1.5ng/dl and you are well and healthy, why would we not consider a hypothyroid condition if at forty-eight years old your TSH increased to 3.5ng/dl, even though 3.5ng/dl is still well within the normal limits for TSH according to laboratory reference ranges? A two-point increase in your TSH can have a major effect on your metabolism and health. Reviewing medical history and looking at previous TSH results as well as observing changes in the body and the development of particular symptoms can be of great benefit in diagnosing a hypothyroid condition.

The greatest wealth is health.

—Virgil

He who has health has hope, and he
who has hope has everything.

—Arabic Proverb

What are T4, T3, reverse T3, and thyroid antibodies?

Free T4 and Free T3: To review, T4 is the major hormone produced by the thyroid gland, and it is the relatively inactive hormone that must be converted to the more-active hormone, T3. Obviously, if low levels of T4 are being secreted by the thyroid gland, there will be less available for conversion to T3. Without enough T3, low metabolism occurs and hypothyroidism exists. Looking at the free T4 and free T3 levels is an additional way to make sure a correct diagnosis is achieved. The *free* levels of these two thyroid hormones simply means that the hormone is not bound to a binding protein. Bound hormones are attached to these binding proteins that make them *inactive* and of no use to the body. Only *unbound* hormones are available for uptake at the cellular level to drive the metabolism. Looking at the unbound levels of both T3 and T4 will provide a more accurate assessment of *active* thyroid levels.

I have observed that many late perimenopausal and postmenopausal women are poor converters of T4 to T3. They may have normal TSH levels as well as normal T4 levels, but they are not converting their T4 to T3 properly. Looking at just TSH (which is more reflective of the level of T4 in the body) will miss this piece of the puzzle.[6] Once female hormones begin to fluctuate during late perimenopause (estrogen dominance and progesterone deficiency) and menopause (both low estrogen and progesterone), the conversion from T4 to T3 in general becomes more sluggish.[7] If the T4 levels are low, a glandular-based endocrine problem exists, which means the thyroid is unable to produce enough of the major hormone T4. This is considered primary hypothyroidism. When T4 levels are normal and T3 levels are low, a conversion problem exists. I will review treatment options later.

Reverse T3 (rT3): If TSH is the gas pedal for thyroid hormones, then reverse T3 is the brakes. Once the TSH rises to stimulate the thyroid gland to produce more thyroid hormones, there must be a way for the body to sense when it has had enough and back off of its production. This is the job of reverse T3. When T4 is secreted into the blood stream, it travels to the specific cells in the body that convert it to the more active form of thyroid hormone, T3, so it can relay to the cells what to do. However, T4 can also convert to a more biologically inactive form called rT3. As I stated above, some rT3 is good and necessary because it is a part of thyroid regulation. However, if T4 is being converted into too much rT3, you can experience all the symptoms of hypothyroidism because T3 levels will then be low. This is not a glandular problem but a metabolic or lifestyle-based one. T4 is converted to rT3 mainly when the body perceives it is under stress and is responding to poor nutrition or lifestyle habits, intentional or unintentional.[8] The proper changes must be made to correct this problem.

Thyroid Antibodies/Autoimmune Thyroiditis: Hypothyroidism is more unique to women than men and is often associated with a genetically inherited autoimmune response. The presence of thyroid antibodies is similar to an allergic response when the immune system overreacts and attacks a foreign invader. The difference, though, is that when thyroid antibodies are present, it is not a foreign invader that it is attacking but the body's own cells. The antibodies bind to the thyroid gland, causing inflammation, which can initially cause an excess of thyroid hormone (hyperthyroid) and eventual destruction of the gland (hypothyroid). The antibodies may also bind to the circulating thyroid hormones and make them unavailable for uptake by the cells. Hashimoto's disease is the most common example of autoimmune thyroiditis and hypothyroidism. In *Hormones, Health, and Happiness*, Dr. Hotze says allergies and hypothyroidism traffic together. He has found that 28 percent of his female allergy patients have the disease, which is much higher than the general population.[9] Testing for food and environmental allergies would be a good idea if thyroid antibodies are present.

Traditional medicine has no real answer as to why people become ill with autoimmune disorders, and autoimmune thyroiditis is no exception. Therefore, if there is no clear underlying cause, then it is hard to treat. However, a number of holistic health-care providers suggest possible triggers of this autoimmune response. The following list gives you an idea of the different situations many holistic providers, such as myself, believe contribute to such an autoimmune response: severe stress (physical and emotional) for a prolonged period of time; bacterial infections; systemic yeast; iodine deficiency; oxidative stress (not enough antioxidant intake); nutrient deficiencies; gluten sensitivity; artificial sweeteners, especially aspartame (Equal, which is metabolized to the toxic substance formaldehyde) and sucralose (Splenda, which is chlorinated table sugar and part of the halide family); and a weakened immune system caused by the abuse of drugs or the presence of other toxic chemicals in the system from prolonged exposure to environmental toxins, chronic inflammation, heavy metal toxicity, and bio and neurotoxins.

I find that once someone tests positive for thyroid antibodies, they will usually continue to test positive. However, working on the immune system and ridding it from some of the infections, toxins, nutrient deficiencies, and so on can greatly decrease the number of antibodies and allow the disease to be treated with the proper thyroid hormones without as much interference from the antibodies. I have witnessed women with thyroid antibodies anywhere from the high one hundreds to the thousands. Trying to balance the thyroid hormones with high antibody levels is like trying to catch a greased pig. The antibodies are out of control, and thyroid levels are all over the place. However, once serious work is done on the immune system by working on improving adrenal function, balancing hormones, taking food allergens out of the diet, reducing inflammation in the body, and correcting nutrient deficiencies, antibodies usually decrease considerably, and thyroid levels begin to stabilize, making treatment less frustrating for the provider and more effective for the client.

How is hypothyroidism treated?

First, you have to know where the problem lies. Doing all of the recommended tests in this chapter is a start. If there is an autoimmune problem, working on the immune system and ridding it of some of the infections, toxins, nutrient deficiencies, and inflammation, as stated above, can greatly decrease the number of thyroid antibodies and allow the disease (hypothyroidism) to be treated with the proper hormones with less interference. Finding a health care provider that has experience in reviewing these different angles is essential.

If there is a glandular problem or a conversion problem, then treating with the proper hormone(s), T4, T3, or both, and balancing the system properly using the combination of history, laboratory results, and clinical symptoms is necessary. Sustained-release T4 preparations are readily available at almost any pharmacy and are very effective in treating hypothyroidism. However, the commercially available T3 (Cytomel®) is an immediate-release thyroid hormone, with almost 95

*Just because you are not sick
doesn't mean you're healthy.*

—Author Unknown

percent being absorbed within four hours. Therefore, it does not sustain a consistent therapeutic level throughout the day as is desired.[10]

In order to maintain good therapeutic levels with this particular medication, smaller amounts of the hormone must be taken several times throughout the day. If you are able to do that, fine. However, I find compliance to be a problem, and patients experience too many highs and lows. Using a compounding pharmacist to compound an extended-release capsule or tablet is the best way to achieve correct, daily therapeutic T3 levels. Compounding can also offer the purest, most precise dosing for each patient whereas commercial preparations are only available in specific, predetermined dosages. Also, commercially available hormones may contain things such as fillers, dyes, and other ingredients that may be potential allergens. Your holistic health-care provider will always have one or several reliable compounding pharmacies at his or her disposal for tailor-making your thyroid hormones to meet your specific needs. They can do the same with BHRT.

What are some other factors responsible for a hypothyroid condition?

Thyroid-Binding Globulin (TBG) and Female Hormones: Thyroid-binding globulin is yet another reason for low thyroid symptoms. TBG is a protein that can attach itself to circulating thyroid hormones. When this happens, the hormone is bound, not unbound as we talked about earlier, and unavailable for uptake by the cells. Female hormonal imbalance, especially estrogen dominance, is one of the major reasons for an increase in TBG. Dr. Hotze states, "

> Estrogen dominance causes the liver to produce increasing levels of thyroid-binding globulin (TBG), a protein that has a strong attraction to circulating thyroid hormones. When TBG latches on to a thyroid hormone, the hormone is no longer free to enter into the cells and be used for metabolic reactions.[11]

He says further that even under ideal circumstances, only about .05 percent of the thyroid hormones circulating in the blood stream are actually unbound and available to the cells. The remainder is bound to

TBG and other blood proteins. Balancing female hormones to arrest the estrogen dominance is essential in keeping circulating levels of TBG down and the thyroid hormones working properly.[12]

Heavy Metals: Although I talk about the subject of heavy metals in my chapter on toxicity, I will mention them here. Heavy metals are a major cause of chronic illness, including thyroid disorders. Dr. Brownstein states in *Overcoming Thyroid Disorders* that nearly 100 percent of his clients with autoimmune disorders test positive for heavy metal toxicity and a large number (greater than 80 percent) with chronic illness, including thyroid disorders, have elevated levels of heavy metals in their systems.[13] Although this may be only one of several reasons, exposure to toxic metals such as mercury, cadmium, lead, arsenic, and nickel predispose the immune system to malfunction and create a resistance to thyroid hormone in the body. Detoxifying and chelating heavy metals from the system almost always improves this resistance situation, allowing a patient's medication to work more effectively, possibly to be lowered, or stopped altogether (see chapter 6 on toxicity, which explains the chelating process).

Iodine Deficiency: It is estimated that over 35 percent of the world's population (almost two billion people) has an iodine deficiency.[14] The thyroid gland must have sufficient amounts of iodine present to make thyroid hormones. Women with low levels of iodine are more prone to develop an enlarged thyroid gland (goiter). As a matter of fact, T4 and T3 molecules each carry four and three iodine molecules, respectively.[15]

Since we live in a world where food and soil can be poor in iodine, perhaps it is possible that a condition perceived as a thyroid problem could be nothing more than an iodine deficiency. I must say that checking for and ruling out iodine deficiency with a twenty-four-hour urine collection may save one from having to take thyroid medication in the first place. However, optimizing iodine levels is important even if thyroid hormone is necessary. It is worth the time and inconvenience for the twenty-four-hour urine collection and iodine test.

Although this subject was not covered in chapter 1 on hormones, iodine deficiency has also been linked to breast cancer in women and is the leading cause for intellectual deficiency in the world.[16] Those are two other very important reasons to make sure iodine levels are optimal.

Please note that iodized salt is insufficient for maintaining proper iodine levels. The amount of iodine in salt may be sufficient to prevent a goiter, but it is not enough to support the rest of the body's needs.[17]

Conclusion

I believe that ordering the proper tests, paying attention to present and past medical and laboratory history, assessing hormone status, nutritional intake and stress level, and working to properly correct the true underlying problems and deficiencies will greatly benefit the metabolic health of any client.

Chapter 4

❦

Digestion and the Intestines

If I could get every person in America (man, woman, and child) to read just one chapter of this book, this one would be it. Many holistic health-care providers have for years postulated that the majority of disease processes begin in the intestines, and I also believe that to be so true. Personally, I not only have a strong genetic history of digestive and colon diseases but have also experienced digestive and intestinal problems.

A Personal Story

Around late perimenopause, I developed chronic laryngitis. After several tests and scopes, it was determined that I had gastroesophageal reflux disease (GERD). In short, this is a disease where the acids of the stomach flow backward into the tube leading from the mouth to the stomach (esophagus), which creates inflammation. This situation was occurring to the degree (mostly at night while I slept) that it was literally burning my vocal cords, causing the chronic laryngitis. During that time, my life was full of stress because my mother had had a stroke and was placed in a nursing home. I am sure a lifetime of improperly digested food and development of unhealthy intestines had a great deal to do with developing this condition, as well as the hormonal imbalances I was experiencing at this time of late perimenopause.

In any case, it all culminated at once, and my stomach and intestines were a mess. Thus began my quest to learn as much about this disease and its causes as possible. What I found has not only eliminated the problem but has also tremendously changed my life and health in many other positive ways. I also know that it can and will change and improve the overall general health of any individual if he or she will make it part of his or her daily routine to take good care of the digestive system and the intestines. Therefore, I would like to share with you the most important lessons about digestive health I have learned.

Again, I continually mention the poor nutritional value of our food and the lack of nutritional intake by the majority of Americans. Although that is a large part of the problem, I won't go there in this book. However, I will attempt to explain how the intestines can get so unhealthy, how it affects the rest of the system, and can be the beginning of all types of disease processes. Also, I will give you some suggestions of how to make sure you are doing the correct things to prevent an unhealthy digestive tract and ward off problems that can be a result of intestinal and colon distress. Again, I will emphasize *preventative* measures.

The digestive system begins at the mouth and ends at the rectum. Everything else in between (the stomach, small and large intestines) is all a part of the digestive system too. The main purpose of digestion is absorption—absorption of nutrients that are vital to overall, good general health. If absorption is poor or suboptimal, then so is nutrient status. It doesn't matter if you are spending hundreds of dollars for the absolute best supplements out there; if there is poor absorption, then you are wasting a lot of your hard-earned money. The truth of the matter is the greater part of the nutrients are going in one end and out the other. We nurses call those undigested supplements "bed pan bullets"!

There are a number of issues that can cause digestive problems that we would not be able to cover in just this one chapter. For instance, digestive problems can range from stomach ulcers related to prolonged and stressful situations to Celiac disease, which is a serious food allergy to gluten, as well as gastritis, reflux disease, diverticulosis, constipation, hemorrhoids, gallbladder problems, and a whole spectrum of others. However, the purpose of this chapter is not to explain all of these diseases/problems and how to treat them but how to take care of your digestive system and *prevent* many health problems and diseases, although most of these suggestions can and will be healing to the intestinal system.

Do you have proper waste elimination?

I think most Americans have a misconception about digestive function and the many aspects of the digestive system. Some believe that if they have daily bowel movements and only occasional constipation, their intestines are healthy. Others believe that the absence of heartburn or reflux after eating indicates their digestive systems are in top working order. Likewise, many presume if they are not experiencing gas, all is well. Not so! Anyone who eats the usual three meals per day and experiences less than two bowel movements (some holistic health-care providers would say three) in the same amount of time is in a constipated state. This constipated condition creates toxic fecal matter that remains in the colon and continues to accumulate, causing a condition that results in an imbalance in the population of microorganisms. This situation leads to abnormal fermentation in the small intestines, often resulting in acute or chronic illness.[1]

Undigested carbohydrates ferment, fats turn rancid, and proteins putrefy. The major problem with undigested food particles is that they often pass into the blood stream (leaky gut syndrome) and are deposited in various parts of the body where this waste manifests as health issues such as high cholesterol, calcium deposits, arthritis, food allergies, cellulite, and plaque in the arteries, to name a few. Also, thirty-six different toxins can be produced in the bowels from this undigested fecal matter, only later to be released into the blood stream.[2] It should always be an automatic occurrence that your body eliminates the waste after digestion. If this is not happening, improper digestion is taking place. The optimum scenario is that food is completely digested, nutrients are absorbed into the blood stream, and the waste products are eliminated completely and properly.

Is there a need for digestive enzymes?

We all know well that when we were young, we could practically eat anything and everything and never seem to have any digestive issues. In our youth, our digestive enzyme banks are full. However, as we age, the years of bad dietary choices tend to catch up with us. Digestive enzymes are depleted, and optimum digestion goes by the wayside.

In order to change, we must be sick
and tired of being sick and tired.

—Author Unknown

Enzymes are pure proteins that are derived from food and made by the body, and they must be present for all biochemical processes. Without enzymes our bodies cannot function. Simply put, enzymes are essential to survival. Not only do we need enzymes for all bodily functions, but we also must have plenty of enzymes for proper digestion and absorption of our foods and nutrients. Dr. DicQie Fuller in *The Healing Power of Enzymes* states, "Enzymes must be present before any chemical reaction can take place. Even vitamins, minerals, and hormones cannot do their jobs without enzymes."[3] She further explains that even "nutrition cannot be explained without describing the vital role played by enzymes."[4] For a moment, I want to focus on the vital role digestive enzymes play in our digestive health.

We are born with the ability to produce enough of these enzymes for proper digestion for many years. However, with the stressful lives we lead in this culture and the quality of our diet in America (lack of raw food consumption with natural enzymes), we deplete our enzymes far faster than we make them and create situations that are disease producing. Dr. Fuller clarifies,

> The importance of proper digestion is mind boggling. Every function must be perfectly synchronized with every other function. When we lack a particular enzyme, vitamin, or mineral, the resulting imbalance causes disease. ... You may think it is too simplistic to conclude that illness is caused by inadequate digestion, but I am convinced this is true.[5]

Clinically, it appears that many women are already showing signs of enzyme deficiency in their early forties or sooner. Further, if a virus or illness is contracted or an emotional crisis encountered, then there is the possibility of enzyme bankruptcy. With this enzyme deficiency comes undigested food being deposited along the intestinal lining, which can eventually lead to poor nutrient absorption and thus a plethora of other unpleasant situations that follow. Although it is recommended that you eat several servings of raw fruits and vegetables each day, even doing so only provides enough natural enzymes to digest that particular food and does not provide the adequate *deposit* of enzymes needed for a surplus. Although this book is written for women, digestive enzyme therapy is essential for men too. Even children in poor health or who are obese would greatly benefit from enzyme therapy.

It is well known that a whole new generation of disease processes is emerging in the young, especially diabetes, obesity, and heart disease, which are directly related to poor dietary habits, lack of digestion, and lack of absorption of essential vitamins, minerals, and nutrients. If, secondary to poor dietary habits, aging, stress, and other factors not already mentioned above, digestive enzyme therapy is highly recommended as part of your supplement and nutritional program, how much more beneficial would it be if enzyme therapy was taken for prevention purposes?

Digestive enzymes work in the intestines helping to support digestion, a healthy colon, and increased absorption of nutrients, but these enzymes also have a positive effect on the entire system. Some additional benefits that may be noted, but are not widely attributed to natural plant enzyme therapy are: increased energy; gallbladder support; a decrease in food allergies, ulcers, diarrhea, constipation, and yeast in the system; good acid/alkaline balance; glucose control; detoxification; healthy cholesterol and triglyceride levels; reduction of free radicals; reduction of inflammation and thus, support of the joints, muscular, and cardiovascular systems; boost in the immune system; support for normal circulation and blood-clotting factors; support for the nervous system; enhanced brain activity; helps balance hormones; helps support normal weight and reshape the body; and decreases the rate of aging. Wow, now that is a list of very positive benefits that everyone can appreciate! A more detailed explanation of many of the above benefits can be found in Dr. Fuller's book, *The Healing Power of Enzymes* (as mentioned above), which I highly recommend as a *must read*. Any woman who wants to improve her digestive and overall health, as well as the health of her family, will gain much wisdom from this book.

How do you know what kind and dose of enzymes to take?

There is a variety of digestive enzymes available, but for the purpose of this book, nutritional, pharmaceutical-grade, plant enzymes are the recommended choice. These particular enzymes have a broader spectrum of use and are manufactured in a more purified and stable form. These are the enzymes I personally use and highly recommend. Although

But we are citizens of heaven, where the Lord Jesus Christ lives. And we are eagerly awaiting for Him to return as our Savior. He will take our weak mortal bodies and change them into glorious bodies like His own, using the same power with which He will bring everything under His control.

Philippians 3:20–21

other forms of digestive enzymes are available, it is not readily known if they contain contaminants, impurities, or fillers. So for investment purposes, the pharmaceutical-grade, plant enzymes will give you the best value for your money. Know your company and the quality of their products.

Before starting enzyme therapy, I recommend that you take my enzyme test located in the back of this book in appendix II. This test has been developed to give you an idea if enzyme therapy is right for you. It will also give you information about which types of foods (i.e., carbohydrates, proteins, fats, or dairy) you may *not* be digesting properly and will help you with your enzyme selection. I prefer and usually recommend a full-spectrum digestive enzyme that contains all of the particular enzymes that act as a catalyst in chemical reactions that break down (digest) the different food groups by hydrolysis (reaction with water). I call them digestive *ases*. For instance, prote*ase* helps digest protein, amyl*ase* helps digest carbohydrates, lip*ase* helps digest fats, lact*ase* helps digest lactose, cellul*ase* helps digest cellulose, and so forth. However, enzymes are made with varying amounts of each of these *ases,* and you can buy enzymes with higher amounts of a particular *ase* according to your specific need(s). For instance, if the test indicates that you are not digesting proteins well, then a digestive enzyme with higher amounts of prote*ase* would be the most beneficial for you. Or if fats are not being digested, you would need an enzyme with sufficient amounts of lip*ase*. Anyway, a full-spectrum enzyme is a really good place to start. Then, if the full-spectrum enzyme does not contain enough of a particular *ase* to do the job, you can add individual enzymes to it from there, such as protease or lipase.

As far as dosing is concerned, some particular problems or situations may require higher doses of enzyme therapy and should be supervised by a health-care professional. However, using one or two capsules of enzymes for *pre*-digestive purposes does not require supervision and can usually be safely taken before, during, after, or in between meals. Enzymes taken before or during a meal will help the food through the digestive process and deliver the nutrients to the body. Taking enzymes after and in between meals can help with the clean-up process and further assist in keeping the walls of the intestines and colon clean and healthy.[6]

When you begin taking enzymes, the amount needed to do the proper job may initially be higher. As you begin to assist the body in the digestive process, clean up the intestinal system, and restore reserves, your need for digestive enzymes may become slightly less.

Do you have a sufficient supply of good flora in your intestines?

Probiotics are another supplement that I consider to be necessary for a healthy digestive system. For proper digestion to take place (breakdown, absorption, and elimination), intestinal flora (the good bacteria) must be intact and in balance. Many microbes live in your intestinal tract, and it is normal to have trillions of intestinal bacteria. Ideally, it is friendly bacteria that aid in the digestion and immune defense processes. However, many common, everyday things can destroy this delicate balance of good bacteria. Using antibiotics, over-the-counter drugs, steroids, a high-fat diet, sugar and high simple carbohydrate consumption, chlorinated drinking water, and contracting parasites are examples of things that can lead to an imbalance in bacteria (and yeast) and eventually lead to illness. There is no better way to restore and maintain a good balance of healthy flora in the intestines than to take a daily probiotic. Eating a healthy diet that may include live cultures is great, but considering the amount of flora we need, it probably will not be enough for the average woman. I always recommend additional supplementation.

If you have not been on probiotics in the past, I recommend that you start with a double dosing of a high-quality probiotic supplement for several months. This replaces the lost flora in larger numbers and allows the bacteria to colonize. Once colonization has begun, then you may cut back to the normal daily dosing to maintain flora balance according to the particular type of probiotic you are consuming. Also, always double or triple your dosing of probiotics for several months after you have had antibiotics, as antibiotics kill both the *good* and the targeted *bad* flora. This way you are assured that you have restored the flora that was destroyed by the antibiotic use.

Probiotics can be found in your local health food store and are safe for man, woman, and child. They can be purchased in tablet, capsule, powder, or liquid form. I prefer a seamless caplet that does not require refrigeration, making it easy and convenient for travel. Also, this type of caplet is not easily broken down by the acids in the stomach, allowing the bacterial flora to be deposited along the intestinal walls where they belong. Stomach acids can destroy most of the good flora before it reaches the intestines in most other forms. However, I believe any amount of good flora is better than none, so do your best to add whatever is available to your daily regimen. This supplement will offer unbelievable benefits for your intestines and immune function.

Should you do bowel cleanses?

Sometimes it is necessary to do an intestinal cleanse. Taking digestive enzymes between meals can do this gently. However, there may be other occasions when a good digestive cleanse is necessary. We live in a world today where international travel is commonplace. Picking up parasites, worms, bacteria, and intestinal viruses from foreign countries is easy to do and happens often. Even in America it is easy to acquire parasites, and again, other intestinal *bugs* from raw fish, meat, poultry, dirt, contact with pets and animals, contaminated water, and so forth. Most people are not aware of the damage these invaders can cause and how to cleanse the system when infestation occurs.

The thought exists that if you obtain an infection from one of these intestinal *bugs,* your body will go into the defense mode and eventually excrete it and all will be fine. This is not entirely true. Even our sophisticated lab testing may fail to identify whether the culprits have been removed from your body. Take parasites, for instance. They can hide in the body, feast off of cells, and cause damage to tissues and organs. They have been associated with diseases like diabetes, cancer, hypertension, liver dysfunction, tumors, and autoimmune diseases. Other symptoms of parasite infestation may be allergies, anemia and nutrient deficiency, constipation, diarrhea, flatulence, bloating, nervousness, and immune dysfunction.[7] Other nonspecific viruses and bacteria have also been known to hide themselves within normal cells while their effects wreak havoc on the immune system without your knowledge.

Again, I am not here to detail where such microbes come from or specifics of how they hide out but to remind you that we are all exposed to them at some time in our life and probably more often than we would

Sickness is the vengeance of nature
for the violation of her laws.

—Charles Simmons

like to think. Now whether or not your body can expel and rid itself of *all* of these *bugs* is the $64,000 question. However, knowing and having seen the distress and diseases these unpleasant organisms can cause, I do recommend an occasional cleanse; and in particular after international travel, I feel it is necessary to cleanse the intestinal system with a product that helps to detoxify worms and parasites.

Diarrhea-type diseases cause almost three million deaths a year. Most are in developing countries where resistant strains of highly pathogenic bacteria and parasites are emerging.[8] If we are fighting and dealing with resistant super-bugs, antibiotics will be more harmful than helpful. Therefore, a natural product to cleanse the intestines is necessary.

How do bowel movements affect your hormone levels?

Bowel movements play an essential role in hormone balance. Whether you are taking exogenous hormones or not, unneeded hormones are excreted by the kidneys and bowels. Obviously, most women have no problem urinating; however, bowel elimination can be a different story, as we have already discussed. When you are constipated, you will reabsorb those hormones that were to be eliminated back into the blood stream from the colon. This can cause a buildup of certain hormones in the system, thus creating an imbalance in hormones. It is imperative to remember this and take this into account, especially those of you who choose BHRT.

Conclusion

As I mentioned several times, most Americans do not have a proper number of bowel movements on a daily basis and are walking around in a constipated state. This induces an overgrowth of the *bad* or wrong kinds of bacteria in the colon; a clogged colon that can lead to leaky gut syndrome; colorectal cancer; irritable bowel syndrome (IBS); diverticulitis; ileitis; inflammatory bowel diseases, which includes Crohn's and ulcerative colitis; *Helicobacter pylori* (a bacteria that is often associated with stomach ulcers and cancer); and many other intestinal problems.[9] This problem can also lead to hormonal imbalances. Eating a wholesome diet, which includes plenty of fiber from fruits and vegetables, conducting an occasional bowel cleanse, and taking the correct supplements to aid in and properly digest your food and keep the bowels moving appropriately on a daily basis is essential to good intestinal health as well as your overall well-being. When it comes to the digestive and intestinal system, believe me, this is one area where an ounce of prevention is worth a pound of cure!

The problem is not that God hasn't spoken, but that we haven't listened.

—Max Lucado
Let the Journey Begin

Chapter 5

The Adrenal System and Adrenal Fatigue

The word *adrenals* is used loosely. You often hear people talking about the adrenals or making statements to the effect that their "adrenals are burned out" secondary to being fatigued. But do you *really* know just how important your adrenals are and what they must do on a daily basis to help your body function properly and at its best? Everything the adrenals provide and do for your overall general health is amazing.

Women are frequently concerned about cancer, heart disease, gynecological health, and brain health. But the glands that help the body cope with the everyday stresses of life—large, small, or anything in between—and *survive it all* are the adrenals. Most women care about their health. When women encounter a particular health concern, they see a doctor for evaluation. However, how many women specifically see a health-care provider to assess their adrenal function? Or coming from the other side, how many health-care providers assess adrenal health or ever suggest that an adrenal function test is warranted? Very few, and sadly so, considering the number of women who are *stressed out* and totally *fatigued* these days. We cannot live without our adrenals, and once the adrenals cease to function, death is imminent. I know that sounds pessimistic, but it is so true. Therefore, because of the little attention the adrenal glands get in conventional medicine, I hope the information I share in this chapter will bring to light the importance of the adrenal glands and mobilize women to think about and take care of this particular and very important part of their health.

What are the adrenals?

There are two adrenal glands. One gland is located on the top of each kidney. They are approximately the size of a walnut and weigh about as much as a grape. However, don't let the size fool you; they not only affect the function of every organ, gland, and tissue in your body, but they also affect the way you feel and think. They largely determine the amount of energy you have in response to every situation you encounter, whether it be internal or external, good or bad. The hormones that are secreted by the adrenals have an influence on all biological processes taking place in the body. Your ability to ward off chronic illnesses or develop certain kinds of diseases is heavily influenced by your adrenal system. In other words, your adrenal health plays an important role in how healthy you feel and the quality of your life.[1]

The adrenal glands are very complex. They are responsible for producing over fifty different hormones, including cortisol, aldosterone, and dehydroepiandrosterone sulfate (DHEA-S), and are a secondary producer of the sex hormones such as progesterone, testosterone, and the estrogens once ovarian function decreases or at the onset of menopause. The adrenals respond to everyday stressors by secreting the well-known hormone called cortisol. However, cortisol is much, much more than that. One of its most important functions is to regulate your immune system. When your body is producing the proper amount of cortisol, it runs very efficiently. Problems arise, however, when you make too much or too little. Too much weakens the immunity, and too little can result in an overactive immune system that releases histamine and other inflammatory substances, causing allergic reactions and more. Both are very common in today's society with all the stressful situations women encounter on a continued basis. The majority of women under stress start out overproducing cortisol to keep up with the daily demands. This scenario continues day after day, month after month, and year after year, until the adrenals are completely exhausted and cannot bear that heavy burden any longer. Then cortisol levels plummet and hypoadrenia or adrenal fatigue sets in.

What are the effects of hypoadrenia or adrenal fatigue?

There are many symptoms of hypoadrenia or adrenal fatigue. One thing is certain: it is not as easily identifiable as some other diseases or problems, such as high blood pressure or a tumor. Most women I encounter who have adrenal problems look pretty normal. They may not display obvious signs of this condition but live with more fatigue and less of an energetic lifestyle than the average person. Often they will be reaching for soda, coffee, or other caffeinated drinks and quick-energy (sugary and high-carbohydrate) foods just to get through the day. Many of these may even have low blood sugars or hypoglycemia, which makes them crave even more of the high-energy drinks and carbohydrates.[2]

Premenstrual dysphoric disorder (PMDD) and a tumultuous transition to menopause can be caused by adrenal fatigue. As adrenal fatigue worsens over the years, other seemingly unrelated conditions may develop such as frequent respiratory infections, allergies, rhinitis, asthma, frequent colds, hypothyroidism, fibromyalgia, chronic fatigue syndrome, alcoholism, and other autoimmune disorders. Individuals experiencing these issues may strike relatives or acquaintances as being just plain lazy or unmotivated when in reality the opposite is true. They usually must force themselves on a day-to-day basis just to accomplish their normal activities. Before this crisis, they were most likely overachievers and people pleasers.

Largely women's understanding of hypoadrenia is lucid. Most women who have this problem are aware that something is wrong, that their energy level is far below that of most of their peers, but when pressed to expound on the subject, they can come up with few details as to why. The basic cause of adrenal fatigue is stress. This stress can come in many forms, such as physical ailments or illness, psychological and emotional situations, environmental factors, infections, and infectious diseases, to name a few, or a combination of any of these.[3] As stated above, the adrenals rally during times such as these and produce the needed cortisol to sustain normal bodily function; however, this only lasts for a limited amount of time. Eventually, the adrenals become so worn out that production of cortisol subsides. The body tries desperately to recover and at times does so with sufficient rest, but if stressful situations or illnesses chronically place high demands on the adrenal system, recovery is difficult. In a more perfect world where only one stressor happens at a time, our adrenals would usually recover quickly; but in fact, we well know that is never the case. Stress is often constant and multifaceted and impairs our adrenal system.

Stress is poison.

—Agave Powers

Stress is an ignorant state.
It believes that everything is an emergency.

—Natalie Goldberg
Wild Mind

What should you do if you think you have low adrenal function?

Find a holistic health-care provider who is willing to test and work with you. Testing is relatively inexpensive. A saliva test to check your hormones is a simple place to start. Hypoadrenia often involves decreased levels of DHEA-S. DHEA-S is a metabolite of DHEA and the hormone that can convert to the sex hormones in both men and women. If there is little DHEA-S, then there will not be enough of this mother hormone to make the conversion to the sex hormones (see next section). Also, DHEA-S and testosterone levels are good indicators of biological age as well as the measurement of adrenal function. A four-point cortisol test will further indicate whether there is too much or too little cortisol being produced and when. These three tests together will aid the provider in diagnosing hypoadrenia, determining its severity, and how best to proceed with treatment. Last but not least, please refer to Dr. James Wilson's book *Adrenal Fatigue: The 21st Century Stress Syndrome.* His book goes into great detail about this subject and includes an adrenal questionnaire that is well worth the price of the book. It also gives guidance to how this condition may be treated and further assists in lifestyle changes that help restore your adrenal function.

How does late perimenopause and postmenopause affect the adrenal system?

In perimenopause and menopause, testing for sex hormone levels and keeping these levels balanced will certainly support the adrenal glands and their proper functioning. As I stated in chapter 1 and in the above section, the adrenal glands take over the job of producing these necessary hormones after the ovaries have ceased doing so. When this happens, the added stress of having to produce these hormones can fatigue the adrenal system. How long this takes depends on the strength of the individual adrenal system at menopause, but eventually it will happen to a greater or lesser degree. Supporting the adrenals by balancing hormones according to test results will give assurance that you are doing all that you can do to keep the burden manageable. Such hormones as pregnenolone and progesterone appear in the adrenal cascade before they are metabolized to DHEA as well as aldosterone and cortisol. Pregnenolone is the first hormone made from cholesterol and progesterone is the second. By replacing hormones "that occur early in the adrenal cascade lets your body's wisdom choose which other hormones it will make from them, according to your body's needs."[4]

It is impossible for the adrenals to manufacture adequate amounts of sex hormones to sustain optimum health in light of the stressors experienced by most women. The sex hormones such as progesterone, estradiol, and testosterone serve to act as antioxidants that forestall the oxidative damage occurring from high levels of circulating cortisol. This is a key factor in aging. Dr. Wilson states, "By bypassing the very complex and energy consuming steps required of your adrenals to make pregnenolone or progesterone from cholesterol, your adrenals do not have to work nearly so hard to keep your hormone levels adequate." He further adds, "Hormones work together in symphony to perform in the concert of life. Hormones are powerful engineers of body processes and balancing them calls for delicate precision. The timing, the quantity, and the form of hormone used are all critical."[5]

Conclusion

Adrenal fatigue is commonplace in today's society. Considering hormone balance along with integral nutrients to help support and restore adrenal function is warranted. I also recommend working with an expert who will properly test all of your adrenal hormones as well as cortisol levels to assess their level of function and if necessary, properly treat and monitor progress. Additionally, there is nothing more important for adrenal fatigue than rest. Take the time to do it!

How beautiful it is to do nothing,
and then to rest afterward.

—Spanish Proverb

Rest is not idleness, and to lie sometimes on the grass
under the trees on a summer's day, listening to the
murmur of the water or watching clouds float across
the sky, is by no means a waste of time.

—Sir John Lubbock

Chapter 6

❧

Environmental Toxicity

This book of information would not be complete without talking a bit about toxicity. It is no secret that we live in a very toxic world. Every second of every day we are taking in toxins that are accumulating in our bodies at an astounding rate. We continuously accrue toxic substances just by breathing, absorbing them through the skin, ingesting them from our food and water supply, as well as from prescribed and over-the-counter drugs and exposure to radiation from foreign electromagnetic fields (see chapter 8). We have come to the point that even our government has approved use of certain toxic chemicals in our environment. Of the more than seventy-five thousand different toxins registered with the Environmental Protection Agency, only a small fraction have undergone complete and thorough testing to determine if they may cause problems for human health. And many have never been tested at all. What a pity that we are exposed to such a variety of environmental toxins on a daily basis and that the government has somehow come to the conclusion that certain levels of these toxins can be so-called normal or okay. Additionally, the majority of the more than two thousand new chemicals that are being introduced into the environment yearly are not subjected to even a simple test to determine toxicity.[1]

Walter Crinnion, ND, a well-known specialist who treats allergies and chronic health problems caused by environmental chemical overload, states that of 210 environmental toxins tested in individuals in a small study done by the Environmental Working Group (EWG),

91 of the 210 toxic compounds (a tiny fraction of the many chemicals registered for daily use in this country) were found in the average person. Each person tested had an average of 53 chemicals that have been linked to cancer and 62 compounds that have been shown to be toxic to the central nervous system. Compounds that were toxic to the immune system averaged 55 per person, and those toxic to the endocrine system averaged 58. Commonly, these toxins adversely affect a number of systems in the body, making them multitaskers. Further, he notes additional studies show that many of these toxins are passed to babies in utero, and he wonders if this situation could account for the increasing rates in childhood brain tumors, autism, asthma, leukemia, and other problems, such as attention deficit and hyperactivity disorders.[2]

Now one may say that our bodies are made to manage these types of poisons and clear them. Well once again, God did create an incredible system that will handle some toxins and expel them from our bodies. However, we were given a toxin-free environment in the beginning and have contaminated it over the years. Now we are on overload and reaping the consequences! We may be slowly destroying our health, and it doesn't look like the situation will get any better anytime soon. I see and feel that our best option to combat this problem is fourfold: 1. To be educated about and aware of the things that are toxic to us in our environment; 2. Reduce exposure to, ingestion of, and use of products that contain toxins (as best we can) over which we have some control; 3. Detox and chelate on a regular *and* ongoing basis (explained later in this chapter); and 4. Educate our families, friends, and communities on this subject because wisdom and understanding can perpetuate or achieve healthy changes in our society.

What is total body burden?

The total body burden is considered to be the total load of all environmental burdens we carry, such as nutritional deficiencies, stress, heavy metals, and all of the environmental toxins. Unfortunately, as we age, there is a bioaccumulative effect, meaning that the total burden increases as time goes on and the body becomes less efficient in the detoxification process.

The effect that these compounds have on our bodies is a very serious issue. They account for many chronic and sometime acute illnesses.

One of the first symptoms is usually fatigue, but other signs of toxicity include immune disorders such as allergies and asthma, chemical sensitivity, polymorphism (a different or abnormal expression of a gene), and chronic infections or difficulty fighting off infections; autoimmune disorders such as lupus, fibromyalgia, and multiple sclerosis; neurological disorders such as headaches, depression, memory loss, and brain fog; and endocrine system disorders such as obesity, insulin resistance, and diabetes.[3]

It looks as though we will be living with these toxins for quite a long time. As stated above, we definitely need to be aware of and educate ourselves, as well as our families, friends, and communities about the detrimental effects of these toxins. Hopefully that will motivate people to take action and support clean food and environmental clean-up acts. However, in the meantime, with the chronic-type of illnesses that these toxins pro-create, we must learn to the best of our ability how to abrogate the effects of these toxins and keep them cleansed from our system. I cannot emphasize enough how critical this is to human health for *current* and *future* generations!

As I write this book, we are seeing the devastating impact of the earthquake and tsunami in Japan. There has been tragic loss of life, but the biggest threat is still developing with the possibility of a meltdown from the nuclear reactors and the releasing of radioactive isotopes into our environment that could affect *all* life on the planet. Traces of atmospheric radiation have already been detected in several states, and many feel that this is just the beginning.[4] How can we protect ourselves and our families from these types of accidents over which we have no control? Thank heaven, God in His great wisdom *has* provided us with some natural resources that can and will help to detoxify our systems. We just need to learn about and take advantage of them. I will talk about how that is accomplished later, but first let us discuss some specifics about toxins.

Where do toxins hide?

Before I go any further, let me explain how these toxins are hidden and stored in the body. The majority of toxins are stored in fat cells. The larger you are, the more toxins you can store. It is the body's way of protecting itself. As toxins enter the system, they are surrounded and

It is well said that there are two things that should never anger us—those things we can change and those things we can't.

—Bob Coy
Dreamality

engulfed by fat cells to get them out of the blood stream as a protection mechanism. However, because we live in such a toxic environment, as we age, the toxins continue to accumulate. If we do nothing to rid ourselves of these toxins, they can cause illness in many forms. The question we may want to ask ourselves is, "Are we aging quicker or just getting more toxic?"

Some individuals are what I call polymorphic (simplistically, different in their genetic makeup). This genetic disorder causes these people to *hang on* to toxins. In other words, they are able to expel very few of these toxins from their bodies, if any at all. These people may be the ones who get the diagnosis of chronic disorders such as fibromyalgia, multiple sclerosis, autoimmune thyroiditis, and other autoimmune disorders for which the medical community has no answers. If the proper care is not taken, these people usually never get better. In many instances their health continues to deteriorate secondary to the cumulative effect of toxins in their systems. And as we already know, people with a poor immune system can be at a higher risk for all kinds of illnesses, including cancer. I believe it essential that we *all* detoxify on a regular basis, but for these particular people it is even more critical.

The lymphatic system is a very complex system made up of organs (tonsils, adenoids, spleen, and thymus), lymph nodes, lymph ducts, and lymph vessels that transport lymph (the fluid and protein that has basically been squeezed out of the blood plasma) from the tissues to the blood stream.[5] This system has many important functions within the body, and it would take a very long time to explain all that this system is capable of doing. However, one of its most important jobs is to provide immune support.

The lymph system detects, filters, and removes bacteria and other foreign invaders from the blood stream. Just like your kidneys, it is another filtering system that cleanses the blood and takes these invaders out of circulation.[6] Unfortunately, there are so many of them in our present environment that the lymphatic system gets overwhelmed and sluggish. I certainly believe that exercise helps to keep things moving both in the bowels and the lymphatic system. However, you are fighting a losing battle if you are not conscientious to exercise and try to avoid and rid your system of as many of these toxins as possible with whatever resources available. The more you are willing to do, the better.

Where do these toxins originate?

Petroleum Products: Besides electropolution (chapter 8) and pharmaceuticals (chapter 7), as already talked about in this book, a large percentage of our toxins come from petrochemicals. Petrochemicals, phthalates (a particular group of petrochemicals used to make hard plastics soft and pliable and are commonly added to cosmetics), and all of their byproducts, such as dioxin, are known to cause an array of serious health problems, such as cancers and endocrine disruptions. Petrochemicals are in many products that we use on a daily basis. Here are just a few of the more common ways in which we ingest and absorb petrochemicals.

Fruits and Vegetables—contain pesticides.

Meat and Dairy Products—contain chemicals from the petroleum-manufacturing process.

Toothpastes—many contain petroleum products, such as artificial colors and mineral oil.

Cosmetics—perfumes, nail, and hair-care products contain phthalates.

Tampons and Sanitary Pads—made from synthetic fibers, which are derived from petroleum.

Clothing—made from synthetic fibers such as acrylic, nylon, and polyester and coated with formaldehyde finishes. Even natural cotton grown for clothing uses enormous amounts of pesticides and petrochemicals and may be just as hazardous as synthetics.

Solvents—used in industrial supplies such as paints and paint thinners, dry cleaning fluids, and cleaning supplies.[7]

Breast cancer has claimed more lives in the last twenty years than the Vietnam and Korean Wars, World War I, and World War II combined. Cancer in general has risen from 5 to 25 percent in the last one hundred years. Cancer rates for Americans were one in four in 1960. Now it is one in two for men and more than one in three for women. When we have so much exposure to petroleum products and their derivatives, which are considered to be carcinogenic, it is hard not to make some kind of connection to toxicity.[8]

Illness occurs when the body's systems are toxic and out-of-balance. One must treat the body as a whole, rather than a series of parts.

—Hippocrates
(464–370 BC)
Father of Medicine

Stop and think about it; it is amazing how many petroleum products we are exposed to, ingest, and use daily. I usually go about my day never thinking twice about many of these things. I tell you this not to alarm you (although in my opinion, you really do need to be alarmed to the greater degree) but to emphasize the necessity in this day and age to make it a part of your routine to cleanse and detox thoroughly at least once or twice per year. Then take the necessary supplements daily that will help you to continually keep your body cleansed and your immune system working properly.

Heavy Metals: Another category of toxins that cause great harm to our health is heavy metals. There are about seventy friendly trace element metals that are needed in the body to carry out certain functions. For instance, iron is needed to prevent anemia, and zinc is a cofactor in over one hundred enzymatic reactions. Magnesium and copper are other familiar metals that are needed in minute amounts for proper metabolism to occur. Such metals normally exist at low concentrations and are known as trace metals. Heavy metals are trace minerals that are at least five times the density of water. They are stable elements, meaning they cannot be metabolized by the body and are bioaccumulative, as we have previously discussed. Heavy metals can also enter the body by inhalation, ingestion, and skin absorption. When heavy metals enter and accumulate in the body faster than the detoxification process occurs, a gradual buildup of these toxins exists and a state of toxicity transpires.

Four of the heavy metals of most concern to human health are lead (Pb), cadmium (Cd), mercury (Hg), and inorganic arsenic (As). These heavy metals are four of the top six hazards present in toxic waste sites, according to the US Agency for Toxic Substances and Disease Registry. Some of the most common problems associated with heavy metal toxicity are: vascular problems, such as blockages and hypertension; adrenal gland dysfunction, which in turn can decrease production of hormones, decrease sex drive, and aggravate menopausal symptoms; decreased responsiveness of diabetics to their medications; neurological diseases, such as depression, decreased mental acuity, and learning and behavioral difficulties, especially in children; exacerbation of conditions like osteoporosis and hypothyroidism; and damage to the brain, kidneys, and a developing fetus.[9]

What degree of exposure to these substances is considered toxic?

It is not necessary for a high-concentration exposure to toxic metals to be present to produce a state of toxicity in bodily tissues and cause health problems. It is the day-in and day-out exposure to trace amounts of these toxins that is harmful. Such common metal toxins can be found in insecticides, weed killers, fungicides, and antifouling paints (*arsenic*); batteries, pigments, metal coatings, and plastics (*cadmium*); storage batteries, ceramics, plastics, packaging materials, paper, inks, water purification processes, and textiles (*lead*); and amalgam fillings, skin-lightening creams, antiseptic creams and ointments, electrical equipment, polyurethane foam production, household utensils, fish and other organisms (mercury).[10] The same is true of petroleum products. Don't let the *trace exposure* concept fool you. Over a period of time, the buildup of these toxins in the system has majorly adverse effects on your health and the health of your family.

How do you rid the body of toxins?

Chelation and Detoxification: For obvious reasons that were discussed above, removing heavy metals and other toxins from the body safely is a concern of many holistic health-care providers. This can be accomplished with chelation and detoxification therapies. Chelates are special types of complexes where the organic molecules bind to a metal at two or more points, thus creating a strong bond. The term chelation comes from the Greek *chele*, meaning claw. When detoxification of heavy metals is discussed, the process of chelation is necessary to remove these particular types of toxins from the body. This detoxification process needs something that is going to grab or attach itself to the metals, produce stable compounds, and enhance the excretion of the metals from the body.

There is much controversy over this subject because the majority of the time when chelation is mentioned, people immediately think about ethylene diamine tetraacetic acid (EDTA), which involves an intravenous procedure. EDTA is an FDA-approved drug for removing metal ions from the body in heavy metal poisoning. Much evidence concerning this procedure has even been submitted to the FDA to support EDTA's effectiveness in the treatment of atherosclerosis and occlusive vascular disorders by the American Academy of Medical Preventics, but the FDA refused to review the data, although EDTA has a much higher lethal dose than the commonly used heart medication digitoxin, the pain remedy aspirin, or the antibiotic tetracycline![11]

Once again, though, I am not here to argue for or against EDTA, although I certainly would consider it if I had a large-scale metal poisoning or was diagnosed with severe atherosclerosis. EDTA is invasive and can sometimes have side effects. However, I am here to encourage you as individuals to chelate on an occasional basis to keep the toxicity of heavy metals (as well as other toxic substances) cleared from your body for preventative purposes. There are a number of ways that this can be done with over-the-counter supplements rather than EDTA.

Conclusion

There are hundreds of published studies available in medical and scientific journals proving that toxic burden does exist. Each time a new study is published, more and more compounds are added to the list. The question of whether there is a toxic burden has already been answered with a resounding *yes*! The question now is how are these many toxins affecting your daily life? Many would rather equate chemical toxicity with things such as cancer and the more serious health problems, but a great number of the common health complaints today are linked to small amounts of daily toxic exposures.[12] As a health-care professional who strives to promote preventative measures, I believe that is where your focus should lie so that you can work to achieve optimum health in this world in which we now live.

Again, a good holistic health-care provider can point you in the right direction for the different types of chelation and detoxification therapies available for ridding the body of these toxins according to your particular needs. This process will pay great dividends to your overall general health! See appendix I for suggestions. Also, let us not forget the benefits of the MRS 2000 with its ability to soften cellular membranes and assist the body in the detoxification process on an ongoing basis. You will read more about the MRS 2000 and pulsating magnetic resonance therapy in chapter 8.

Conviction is worthless unless it
is converted into conduct.

—Thomas Carlyle

Chapter 7

✿

The Yeast Syndrome

*I*t has been twenty-eight years since Dr. C. Orian Truss's book *The Missing Diagnosis* introduced the world to a yeast-like fungus called *Candida albicans,* which he believed was responsible for a vast number of human ailments and diseases, from depression and hormonal disturbances to allergic reactions and autoimmune disorders. Chronic systemic yeast infections, he believed, may also be a causative factor in diseases such as multiple sclerosis, Crohn's disease, schizophrenia, myasthenia gravis, and lupus.[1]

He eventually found that his symptomatic patients who cultured positive for Candida got much better after treatment with an antifungal. He also noticed that other clinical symptoms, such as headaches and gastrointestinal problems, also improved.[2] Although this subject has also been written about extensively in Dr. William Crook's book, *The Yeast Connection* and has been talked about and debated over and over these past years, I am uncertain that any of this has made much difference in the traditional medical community. Yeast overgrowth, unfortunately, is still not often recognized as a significant risk to one's health. Any yeast problem is usually looked at primarily as a localized invasion, such as oral thrush, a vaginal yeast infection, or a toenail fungus, and treated accordingly.

Part of the skepticism comes from the fact that although *Candida ablicans* may be the cause, it has never been proven to be the culprit, says Dr. Keith Eaton, a leading specialist.[3] Naturopath Harald Gaier, director of medical research at London's Hale Clinic, agrees: "Clearly, other similar organisms such as Candida utilis, Torulopsis glabrata, or even Crytococcus hystolticus may be responsible, or indeed parasites like Giardia lamblia or Blastocytis hominis."[4] Another possible reason for such skepticism is that this yeast lives in every human being, so it makes it impossible to track down or be labeled as a factor in certain conditions. Further, the multiple symptoms it causes can easily be conveniently labeled as other illnesses.

As a health-care provider, I certainly know that the body is highly complex, so looking at a particular problem or set of symptoms and trying to narrow down the exact cause can be demanding at times, to say the least. Then, determining whether yeast is involved or part of the culprit provides an additional challenge. However, clinically speaking, I don't think it has to be that difficult to decipher. There are a large number of symptoms that indicate yeast overgrowth exists. Does that mean if a person has one or two of these particular symptoms that yeast is the issue? No. But don't you think if you have a set of particular chronic symptoms or health problems and you have tried everything else to no avail, it would at least be worth your while to look into the matter? I do, especially if it means you can possibly resolve a number of your health concerns. So let us examine some questions to help you further understand this subject of yeast overgrowth. And once again, I will make some suggestions that will help you to know when the yeast in your system is most likely out of balance, what causes it, and how to keep the yeast stable and in check. Doing so will help prevent breakdown of the immune system and future disease processes that may be initiated by this particular problem.

What is yeast overgrowth?

The body is designed to have a delicate balance of both good bacterial flora and yeast. Like almost everything else in the body, when the balance is gone, problems will arise sooner or later. Again, in God's design, the body is miraculous and can withstand a lot of ill-treatment. It reminds me of an old watch commercial that went something like this: "It takes a lickin' and keeps on tickin'," at least for a while, in spite of the abuse. That all depends on how strong the immune system is initially and how much the yeast has overgrown. The greater the yeast problem, the faster and more furious the symptoms will come.

I have heard it described this way: You should look at our body as an empty barrel when you are born. As you grow and the years pass by, you fill it up with *stuff*. That *stuff* can be *good*, or it can be *bad*. The *bad* can include toxins of all kinds as well as unhealthy foods in your diet. Just because it was put in there five, ten, fifteen, twenty, or twenty-five years ago doesn't necessarily mean that the effects or future effects of some of the bad is now gone. Your body has the ability to get rid of some of the bad *stuff* (as I discussed earlier), but once again, and because of the many environmental toxins and the horrible American diet, there is a continuation to introduce more bad *stuff* into our systems. Further, a certain amount of the bad *stuff* that was introduced years ago is still there also. How much still remains all depends on your own particular immune system and how well it is working, as well as your knowledge of how to assist the body in ridding itself of the bad *stuff*.

Okay, so much about *stuff*. However, I am trying to drive a point here. When you do things to your body that can cause yeast overgrowth or Candidiasis, it continues to increase in the system until one day there is that next straw that breaks the camel's back, so to speak, and symptoms develop. They may be mild at first, but if nothing is done to regain that balance, and more unhealthy substances are put into the system that can further increase the yeast, additional symptoms can occur and magnify the current symptoms. Eventually a disease of some sort will develop. In traditional medical circles, it is unusual that Candida is ever blamed as one of the culprits, and treatment for this condition is not likely to be suggested.

So let's get back to the question, "What is yeast overgrowth?" Short and simply, yeast overgrowth is just that: an overgrowth of yeast in the system that disrupts the naturally healthy balance.

What causes yeast overgrowth?

I believe some of the chief causes of yeast overgrowth are sugar and simple carbohydrate consumption, antibiotics, and prescription and over-the-counter drugs. Let us take a closer look at these subjects.

Sugar: There are a number of articles that talk about sugar consumption and all sorts of data that look at this subject from different demographic angles. However, it is common knowledge that the typical American is addicted to sugar. In 1967, the average American consumed

Insanity: doing the same thing over and over
again and expecting different results.

—Albert Einstein

about 114 pounds of sugar per capita per year. By 2003 that number rose to 142 pounds per capita per year.[5] The United States Department of Agriculture reported 158 pounds per year per person in 1999, 30 percent higher than in 1983 and equivalent to about fifty teaspoons per day.[6]

Unfortunately, regular white sugar is just one component of the total sweetener supply. Corn sweetener consumption increased to seventy-nine pounds per capita in 2003, up 400 percent from 1970. This very steep rise in consumption was largely due to the introduction of high-fructose corn syrup, a low-cost substitute that sweetens the many sugary beverages that Americans seem to crave.[7] Since 1950, soft drink consumption has increased from about eleven gallons per person per year to forty-six gallons per year in 2003. That's nearly a gallon a week per person. This compares to a dismal eight-point-three pounds of broccoli and slightly over twenty-five pounds of dark lettuces (the kinds that are really good for you).[8]

Now add to the sugars other simple-carbohydrate foods such as breads and pastas that may be consumed on a daily basis and it is easy to see that Americans have a serious problem with overeating sugar, whether or not you agree with the above statistics. Regardless of where you get your sugar fix, sugar increases yeast in the system. Yeast thrives on sugar. The higher the yeast in your system, the more you will crave sugar. And the more sugar you eat, the more the yeast will overgrow. It can become a vicious cycle.

Although there are yeast and molds in the air that cannot be avoided, changing your diet to include less sugar is helpful. Moderation is the key according to your activity level. Sugar is nothing more than empty calories, and aside from yeast, a diet high in sugar contributes to obesity, diabetes, osteoporosis, cancer, and heart disease.[9] Complex carbohydrates such as fruits and vegetables should be the place to look for your quick energy needs.[10] The more you get back to a simple diet based on whole foods, the better. Artificial sweeteners should be avoided, as most are toxic to humans and cause DNA strand breaks.[11]

Antibiotics: This was a very interesting subject to research. I found all sorts of articles and information on antibiotics and resistance but not as much about the consumption of antibiotics by Americans (i.e., the amount). Where would we be without antibiotics? I am not against antibiotic use when they are warranted. Antibiotics have significantly contributed to reduction in death rates over the past fifty years. However, the general consumption of antibiotics has increased (with the exception of a slight decrease in the 1990s) during the past fifty years.[12] Researchers suggest that almost one-third of antibiotic prescriptions are questionable, and many believe it is more like 40 to 60 percent. Although many medical providers understand that resistance can cause antibiotics to become a scarce resource and are trying to cut down on the unnecessary use of antibiotics to avoid resistance, often the trend to satisfy patients and give them a quick fix encourages inappropriate prescribing practices.[13] Antibiotics are also needlessly and frequently used to help with common viral infections. Dr. Gary Null states, "Even though 90 percent of all upper respiratory infections are caused by a virus, over 50 percent of the time the patient will come out with a prescription for an antibiotic."[14]

When you take antibiotics, you are not only killing off the disease-causing bacteria that you are trying to get rid of in the body, but you are also killing off the good or helpful bacterial flora that keeps the yeast in check and increases immune function. Taking antibiotics dramatically reduces bowel elimination, kills friendly flora, slows digestion, increases gas and bloating, and causes constipation or diarrhea as well as increases the yeast, most notably Candida, in the gut.[15, 16] Antibiotics can cause fatigue, allergic reactions, and many more harmful things, not to mention that prescription antibiotics are synthetic and are themselves a toxin.

For the majority of women, I do not think that antibiotics in themselves are a huge problem, unless they are used on a long-term basis. Most women I know put off going to the doctor and suffer through most colds, flu, minor health problems, and even more severe illnesses. They are often too busy taking care of everyone else and not taking enough time to care for themselves. I think the real problem lies in not understanding, knowing, or being taught how to negate the effects of antibiotics when and if they are needed and taken. Once you finish reading this chapter, though, you should have better knowledge on this subject.

Over-the-counter and other prescription medications: In 2002, it was reported that the United States spent more than ninety billion dollars a year on prescription drugs alone. That was more than

One person with courage makes a majority.

—Andrew Jackson

1 percent of the entire Gross Domestic Product. Between 1997 and 1999, money spent on prescription drugs grew nearly two hundred times faster than overall national health expenditures.[17] Medco Health, the nation's largest pharmacy benefit manager, says that even money spent on prescription drugs to treat children (infants to nineteen years old) for such things as asthma, high cholesterol, gastroesophageal reflux disease, and hypertension soared by 10.8 percent in 2009, which was more than triple the increase in that of senior citizens. These statistics do not take into account all of the money spent on over-the-counter drugs (which are not included in insurance plans) for such things as colds, flu, insomnia, headaches, pain, and the list goes on and on.[18] Many Americans take daily prescription medications and also use their fair share of over-the-counter products for various aches, pains, and other particular conditions. As I usually try to make very clear, I am not here to condemn anyone for their choices. I am just here to present the facts. One fact is very obvious: the consumption of drugs (prescription and nonprescription) is soaring.

These drugs drastically change the intestinal tract and kill the good flora that keep Candida in check, therefore allowing fungi to quickly take hold and begin multiplying. Candida is a very aggressive fungus and pushes its way into the intestinal lining, destroying cells and brush borders along the way. Brush borders are the microvilli that have the important function of nutrient absorption in the gastrointestinal tract. Once these brush borders are damaged, it is a complex process to restore them, if at all, depending on the amount of damage and the time that has passed. In addition, larger amounts of Candida produce their own toxins, which further irritate and break down the intestinal lining.[19] It is imperative to restore this delicate flora balance and use the proper supplements to reduce inflammation and begin healing the intestinal lining as much as is possible. Your nutrient absorption and overall well-being is largely dependent on this.

How can you tell if you have Candida?

I have provided a simplified Candida questionnaire form in appendix III. This is a good resource to assess your past medical history and symptoms. It is a simple way to check yourself. The higher the score, the worse the condition. Also, if you do not score very high, it doesn't mean that you will not benefit from a good yeast cleanse every now and then. You should assess yourself yearly and especially after any acute illness or development of new symptoms. As I see it, this should be an ongoing effort in the world in which we live today. Dr. Abraham Hoffer, a physician in the field of orthomolecular psychiatry, has used a yeast protocol successfully on many of his clients. He believes that one-third of the world's population is affected by Candida.[20] That is an enormous number of people walking around with a yeast problem! And most likely they will never be treated.

Numerous health problems have been associated with the overgrowth of yeast in the system. It can be something as minor as occasional indigestion or irritable bowel syndrome to more serious diseases such as multiple sclerosis, lupus, leaky gut syndrome, psoriasis, eczema, and all sorts of food allergies and chemical sensitivities. Other symptoms may include, but are not limited to: frequent infections; fatigue; trouble concentrating; poor coordination; muscle weakness; joint pain; mood swings; depression and other psychiatric disorders such as anxiety, panic attacks, and personality changes; dry mouth or throat; catarrh (inflammation of the nasal passages with increased mucus production); pressure above the eyes or ears; frequent headaches; pain in the chest; shortness of breath; dizziness; easy bruising; asthma; vaginal burning or itching; vaginal discharge and infections; frequent urinary tract infections; premenstrual syndrome; fibromyalgia; weight gain; and difficulty getting pregnant.[21]

How is yeast or Candida treated?

There are a number of ways to treat yeast, and treatment will depend on the severity of the yeast problem. Obviously, it will have to be with some sort of antifungal medication or supplement that helps reduce yeast in the system. Just as treating any other infection, the question to consider is, do you need the big guns or will a water pistol do? Depending on the score of the questionnaire and the patient's personal history, I can usually make that judgment. I like to work with my patients and give them the option of going with a prescriptive antifungal or starting with more natural, nonprescriptive-type antifungal treatments. If I believe the yeast to be really bad, I may recommend a combination treatment which includes starting with a prescriptive antifungal (short-term) and then switching to a more natural cleanse. Your holistic health-care provider will know what to do and be able to help you make the correct choice for your particular condition, if it warrants seeing a professional. If not, the questionnaire and a common-sense review of your medical history will do. I would love to think I or other health-care professionals are the only who can make the diagnosis. Fortunately for you, it doesn't always take the likes of us to figure it out.

Up until this point, I have avoided listing particular supplements or giving specifics about what to take since each individual is different and has different needs. However, I did say above that by the end of this chapter, I wanted you to know what to do and how to avoid yeast overgrowth, so I certainly don't want to leave you hanging. What I really desire is to inform you of a few simple things (besides changing your diet) you can do on your own to balance the yeast in your system and *prevent* yeast overgrowth in the future.

You have already read chapter 4, "The Digestive System and the Intestines." Some of my suggestions in that chapter will directly relate to helping keep yeast at bay and will be reiterated here:

1. **Digestive Enzymes**: Enzymes help in the process of breaking down food properly, which aids in reducing the environment in the intestines that breeds bad bacteria and allows yeast to overgrow. If yeast is a problem, this can be added daily regardless of age.

2. **Probiotics**: Probiotics colonize and increase the amount of healthy flora in the gut to keep yeast in check and bad bacteria down. They further support the digestive process, which in turn increases the immune function. This is essential to *all* on a daily basis. If it is necessary to take antibiotics or steroids, double or triple your probiotic use and continue for at least two months after completion of the medication. Then you may resume a maintenance dose. For the very best results, probiotics should be taken at least one hour before or one hour after meals.

3. **Yeast Cleanse**: A yeast cleanse once or twice a year is a preventative measure, since we know that yeast overgrowth is a problem we need to continually assess for and

When we lose the right to be different
we lose the privilege to be free.

—*Charles Evans Hughes*

treat. However, a yeast cleanse is always recommended immediately after finishing a course of antibiotics or any steroid medication. If you have a holistic health-care provider, he or she can help you determine whether you will need a prescriptive antifungal or if an over-the-counter supplement is best. Seek the assistance. Anything that is attempted to avoid yeast overgrowth will be valuable to your overall general health. Whatever you choose to take, you should consult a physician or health-care provider if you are on any other medication(s) to make sure there are no negative interactions.

A few of my over-the-counter favorites for cleansing yeast include:

a. Results RNA ACS (Advanced Cellular Silver): This powerful nano silver has been proven capable of killing an array of disease-causing organisms. It oxidizes the cell wall of gram-positive and gram-negative bacteria as well as naked viruses and fungi, all without damaging human tissue. ACS is dispensed in a spray form and highly absorbable, so you don't have to worry about its efficacy since it does not have to go through the intestinal tract. It is very effective for those whose yeast problem is most likely a systemic issue.[22] This is a nonprescriptive product but must be purchased from a clinic or medical provider. (See appendix I.)

b. Protease: Protease is an enzyme that digests proteins. However, protease has long been used by holistic health-care providers as an effective treatment for Candida. It also can break the cell wall of fungi and serve to reduce yeast in the system.[23] Protease should be taken in between meals for it to be most effective in a yeast cleanse.

c. Caprylic Acid: This is a naturally occurring fatty acid that has been found to have antifungal activity. Some professionals think that Caprylic acid is just as good as Nystatin, which is a prescriptive antifungal that works in the gut.[24]

d. Citrus Seed Extract: Another natural antifungal that discourages the growth of Candida in the intestines. It is also effective against Giardia and other intestinal parasites.[25]

e. Garlic: For centuries, garlic has been used for medicinal purposes for such things as a remedy for pneumonia to snake bites. It is also widely documented as an antifungal agent. It is available in odorless preparations.[26]

f. Goldenseal: A perennial herb that has been used by Native Americans for a wide range of medicinal purposes and to fight infections. It has been found to be effective against a number of organisms, including Candida .[27]

e. Aloe Vera: The gel from the Aloe Vera plant has demonstrated to have biological activity against common bacteria and fungi like *Candida albicans.*[28]

Prescriptive antifungals include products such as Diflucan (fluconazole), Nizoral (ketoconazole), and Nystatin (ketoconazole prototype). I have found the first two are more effective for systemic yeast infections. Nystatin works well in the gut only. Again, your holistic health practitioner can help make the judgment about whether your symptoms point toward a systemic or intestinal infection and the type of treatment needed.

Conclusion

Changing your diet to avoid overloading the system with simple carbohydrates and sugars, only taking necessary medications, and using more natural products and preparations for colds and flu will help keep yeast in balance in the system. Further, adding digestive enzymes and probiotics to your daily regimen and learning how to assess and treat yeast overgrowth when necessary and on an ongoing basis will develop your skills in keeping yeast in check and your immune system strong and healthy. Regardless of the criticism for working outside the customary norms from the traditional medical community, many of my clients have been totally, but pleasantly, surprised by how much their health improved by treating the often-overlooked health problem called Candida.

Originality is simply a pair of fresh eyes.

—Thomas W. Higginson

*Originality implies being bold enough
to go beyond accepted norms.*

—Anthony Storr

Chapter 8

Pulsating Magnetic Resonance Therapy and the MRS 2000

I know many of you have not heard of this therapy or been exposed to it previously. However, because I have had and seen so much success with this therapy in my practice as well as other health-care practices in my local area, I wanted to include a short chapter on the subject. Magnetic resonance therapy is probably one of the best and most effective, noninvasive treatment modalities to come along in quite some time. It is very beneficial for health and healing, and I want to introduce this therapy to you and explain what it is, how it works, and its many uses today by individuals for health and wellness.

What is pulsating magnetic resonance therapy?

Currently, energy medicine is the newest and most cutting edge alternative treatment, and pulsating magnetic resonance therapy (PMRT) is no exception. Despite the large amount of research on this subject, magnetic field therapy remains practically unknown to Americans today outside of patients who have used this healing modality for fractures and wounds. PMRT is a very young but vast science and a different form of therapy than has previously been available.[1] It is not meant to be a miracle but a wonderful modality used for accelerated therapeutic purposes as well as for general health and wellness. PMRT is a very efficient and simple therapy method. By influencing the client with either general or local pulsating magnetic fields, cellular functions can be improved considerably. It is quantum physics at its best, and it would be impossible for me, a layperson, to explain this science. However, if you are really interested in learning the basic principles of quantum mechanics in health and disease, you may want to read the book *Magnetic Resonance Stimulation, Using the Field to Maximize Your Health* by Joel Carmichael, DC.

It is common knowledge that we are electrical beings. Every cell in our body, whether in tissue or bone, has a certain electrical potential. Once that electrical potential is gone from all of our cells, we are dead. Somber thought. However, many people walk around every day with very little of that much-needed electrical potential in their cells secondary to disease, bad diet, low immune function, stress, or all of the above. The various unhealthy aspects of our lives (many which I have discussed in this book) act as invisible energy robbers. They cause permanent stress and diminish the energy supply to our cells. In addition, our exposure to *electromagnetic smog* (electropollution) with its abnormal foreign frequencies interferes with the muted resonance of the cell. This in turn reduces the voltage potential and affects our vitality. Energy medicine observes that disturbed cellular function is the basis of all disease. The goal with PMRT is to restore the energy flow and balance *in* and *through* the body.[2]

Please be aware that PMRT (which produces electromagnetic fields) is not the same as stationary magnetic therapy. To be therapeutic, a magnetic field must change to have an electrical effect. Regular, stationary magnets that radiate a static, unchanging magnetic field *do not* and *will not* produce electrical fields. You may know of someone who wears a magnetic bracelet, necklace, or other apparatus or has magnetic pads, bandages, or mattresses. Those magnets are static and do not produce the necessary electrical field to have any therapeutic benefit. Dr. Carmichael says:

> Because they have a time-varying frequency, pulsating electromagnetic fields easily produce cell induction (cell membrane ion dissociation) through lower levels without producing cell fatigue. That is, the frequencies and/or amplitudes are dynamic and always changing so the cells do not habituate, or fatigue, to the stimulus. Static magnets produce only one

field strength and no frequency. Cells habituate to that field strength.[3]

So, the static field may eventually do more harm than good. Only pulsating or changing magnetic fields have been shown to have benefit.

Japanese researcher K. Nakagawa evaluated more than eleven thousand human subjects and concluded in large part that Westerners are suffering from a lack of magnetic field, an epidemic of magnetic field deficiency. The human body requires sufficient levels of magnetic energy for optimum health. When lacking, it can manifest itself as chronic illness, and he suggests that possibly fibromyalgia, chronic fatigue syndrome, and other disease processes involving pain and fatigue are really magnetic deficiency syndromes. He has identified the fact that our bodies require sufficient amounts of magnetic energy for optimum health. When you understand the relationship between disease and the lack of energy potential in the cells, as discussed above, you can believe that to be so. Our lifestyles, living conditions, transportation modes, and work environments are such in this day and age that we do not receive adequate exposure to the earth's magnetic field anymore, and all of us could benefit from daily supplemental exposure in the pursuit of wellness and pain-free living.[4]

If you can't see electropollution, is it still harmful?

Besides all of the chemical toxins that we introduce into our bodies, as discussed in the chapter on toxicity, whether intentional or unintentional, electropollution is a significant cause of this decreased cellular energy today. Our bodies are constantly bombarded by electropollution from power lines, transmitters, electrical wiring, video games, televisions, and appliances. These create what we call electromagnetic frequencies (EMFs) that are estimated to be 100 million times greater than they were one hundred years ago. Compounding this problem is the explosion of the wireless technology in use today such as cell phones, Bluetooth accessories, wireless Internet, and the powerful microwave towers that are required for transmission of these devices. This world of pervasive wireless technology emits its own spectrum of EMFs that have damaging effects on living systems. It really doesn't matter anymore whether you

Energy, like the biblical grain of the
mustard seed, will remove mountains.

—Hosea Ballou

use a cell phone, computer, or any of this technology; you and everyone else are exposed to this dangerous radiation from the proliferation of this wireless technology. Sorry, but there is nowhere to hide anymore! Just because you can't see it doesn't mean it won't hurt you.

Research on this body of science acknowledges that EMFs are presently the greatest threat to our health and well-being. Hundreds of studies have shown and concluded that EMFs have harmful effects on our immune system, enzyme syntheses, endocrine system, nervous system, learning, moods, and behavioral patterns. All aspects of life can potentially be damaged by electroplating, and many health problems have been associated with EMFs, including various cancers (especially eye, ear, brain, and leukemia), miscarriages and birth defects, learning disabilities, chronic fatigue, headaches, stress, nausea, heart problems, and insomnia. Whatever your thoughts may be about this wireless world in which we live, whether you can see it or not, it does affect our health and the health of our families. These frequencies are unfamiliar to our bodies and are perceived as dangerous, foreign invaders. Dr. Robert O. Becker, author, medical researcher, twice Nobel Prize nominee, and expert on electromagnetic radiation, is particularly concerned about electropollution. He says, "I have no doubt in my mind that at the present time, the greatest polluting element in the earth's environment is the proliferation of electromagnetic fields."[5] He even considers this problem to be worse on a global scale than warming and the increase in chemical elements in the environment. Wow, that's some statement to think about!

How can PMRT help?

There are a number of different pulsating magnetic units on the market, but I personally use the MRS 2000. (The new, updated unit is called the iMRS.) It is German made and has been used in Europe and Russia with tremendous success. Many households in Europe and around the world own one of these units for personal and family use. Unlike America, where traditional medicine treats by probing, prodding, injecting, and poisoning, other countries are and have been far ahead of the United States in utilizing more holistic and natural health treatment alternatives. And the MRS 2000 is no exception. Millions of these units are in use on a daily basis in Europe and around the world. It is the number one pulsating magnetic resonance unit sold in the world today. The MRS 2000 also has a light sound unit that attaches and is useful for rest and relaxation and in certain conditions, such as depression, attention deficit disorder (ADD), and attention deficit/hyperactivity disorder (ADHD). Pulsating magnetic fields have been used to help in many situations. Below are just a few of the conditions for which it may be of benefit:

Removing waste and toxins in the body	Stress relief
Reducing inflammation	Migraine headaches
Enhancing sports performance	Neuralgias
Pain relief from injury or arthritis	Improve sleep patterns
Increased energy	Wound healing
Bone healing (broken)	Increase bone density
Increased oxygen in the tissue	Regeneration of vascular tissue
Increased lymph drainage	Chronic fatigue
Degenerative spine and joint tissue	ADHD, ADD, panic attacks
Depression	Immune deficiencies
Fungal infections	Improved respiration
Improved blood circulation in capillaries	Overall well-being/relaxation[6]

I have used the MRS 2000 unit and PMRT in my clinic now for over four years. I have seen the benefits that my clients have received from this type of therapy. I have personally used it to decrease the healing time in fractures and deep ulcers, decrease back and shoulder pain, get bowels moving in chronically ill patients, improve sleep, improve plantar fasciitis and other foot pain, reduce pocket depth in gums, reduce inflammation, and treat myalgia and muscular soreness as well as chronic pain. My colleagues have been equally successful using this unit to reduce pain and increase energy in fibromyalgia patients, improve sports performance and treat sports injuries, relieve migraine headaches, improve bone density in osteopenia and osteoporosis patients, improve blood flow and oxygenation, and improve the symptoms of ADD and ADHD, to name a few.

Conclusion

Simply said, this is how PMRT works. Humans and animal organisms consist of a large number of cells that function electrically. The cell membrane is where the resonant effect can take place. All *healthy* cells have an inherent oscillation with a certain frequency and amplitude.[7] If there is no electrical potential left in a cell, the cell is no longer viable and cannot recover to a certain potential that is necessary for normal cellular function. Diseased or damaged cells have an altered rest potential. If the ions (electrically charged particles surrounding the cells) move into an area of pulsating magnetic fields, they will be influenced by that rhythm of pulsation and be revitalized. When an ion exchange takes place, it is also responsible for the oxygen utilization of the cell. PMRT can dramatically influence ion exchange at the cellular level and greatly improve oxygen utilization.[8] Increased oxygen equals ionic migration (movement of potassium, chloride, calcium, and protein through the cell wall), thus enhancing cellular energy. In this environment, healing can take place and the potential for optimum health can be restored.

Pulsating magnetic resonance is an amazing therapy and has the potential to restore the body compromised by many different and unhealthy circumstances. Research has proven that low-energy pulsating fields can produce remarkable positive changes within the body.[9] Olympians in Europe, as well as other professional athletes

*All good things which exist are
the fruits of originality.*

—John Stuart Mill

and individuals, have used this therapy for years with proven success. The MRS 2000 is a wellness unit. It doesn't know if you are ill or well. It doesn't know what parts of the body need to be revitalized; however, its pulsating magnetic fields can help the body to restore its own energy potentials, reduce inflammation, and begin healing itself. If you are suffering from a chronic condition, chronic pain, or any of the conditions mentioned above or just want to de-age inside, it is one of the best health and wellness units and adjunctive or alternative healing modalities around. Do your own research. Again, Dr. Joel Carmichael's book, *Magnetic Resonance Stimulation, Using the Field to Maximize Your Health*, can explain in further technical detail how pulsating magnetic resonance is beneficial and needed in our environment today.

If you would like more information about this particular therapy and how it may benefit you, please e-mail my office at: judyponsford@ yahoo.com, or call (303) 805-5466.

Chapter 9

꙳

Money and Health Principles

At this point in the book, I am sure you weren't expecting a talk about money. You are most likely thinking, *What does money have to do with hormones and health?* Well, I am not really here to give you a finance lesson, per se, but mostly to encourage you to make wise choices with your money when it comes to your health. What you do now for your health will pay dividends in the years to come.

At the writing of this book, the economy is awful. We are all suffering to some degree and trying desperately to make our money go further in this down-turned economy. Hopefully the economy will improve soon, but if you are suffering from some ills, it really doesn't matter about the economy. What matters is that you get help and you get the help you need to improve your quality of life. It's like the credit card commercial—your health is priceless! The amount of money you spend on improving your health is worth every penny. It truly is pay now or pay later.

I have seen a trend in recent years where insurance companies are raising their premiums to the point that individuals are opting for plans with higher deductibles. Therefore, a larger portion or all of preventative health-care costs must come out of pocket. Even if you have the most wonderful insurance plan in the world, holistic and alternative health care, nutritional supplements, and compounded hormones are usually not covered. So where does that leave us? It leaves us pulling from the bottom of our pockets to pay for these preventative measures that we need for optimum health.

Through this entire book, everything I have written about has been geared to the prevention of disease. Yes, *prevention* is the key word. Prevention means to avoid the occurrence of something that is perceived to have a negative outcome. It should be your desire to prevent negative outcomes that could possibly occur in the future by taking proper precautionary measures. In other words, you must not neglect the important practices that must be put into place today so that you are confident you have done all you can do to make your future brighter. That lesson can apply to many things in your life, but at this moment I would like to place emphasis on your health.

Prevention (from illness) is just that—doing the correct things now that will also provide some favorable health benefits in the future, although at times it may seem unnecessary. The purpose of this chapter is to encourage you to take those necessary precautionary measures *now*. Don't wait! Can I promise you that nothing bad is ever going to happen to you? Can I promise that you are never going to get cancer or some other disease or that you will live a long and healthy life with minimal problems and then simply pass gently and quietly? Wow, we all wish that were the case! However, the answer to the question is no. We have no guarantees in life concerning our health. Nonetheless, that should never stop us from trying to the best of our ability to do what has been proven time and time again to help in certain situations, and that includes all of the hormonal and nutritional therapies that we know will improve our health and help us *prevent* disease. Now that brings me back to the topic of money. You well know that quality nutrition and compounded hormones cost money. Even over-the-counter drugs and co-pays for prescribed synthetic drugs are expensive. However, if you are serious about your health and desire to optimize the efficiency of this marvelously God-created machine known as your body, then budgeting for some out-of-network provider care and quality supplements is essential.

I personally spend a lot of my hard-earned dollars on compounded hormones and supplements each month. If I didn't truly see the benefits and believe they are and will in the future make a difference in my health and quality of life, I wouldn't take them or spend my money on them. After many years of taking and testing different products and product lines, I have found that the best quality and most effective

Cherish your health: If it is good, preserve it.
If it is unstable, improve it. If it is beyond
what you can improve, get help.

—Author Unknown

Begin to be now what you will be hereafter.

—William James

supplements are usually the most costly ones (unfortunately). However, at this point in my life, you could not pry any of them out of my hands. In essence, you get what you pay for. Since nutritional supplements are not FDA regulated, it is sometimes difficult to know which way to go when it comes to choosing brands. Nevertheless, a little research on your part can reveal a great deal about a company and the quality of nutrients it manufactures. Make it a goal to do your homework before you shop and purchase quality.

Since I suspect a number of you have sensitivities and food allergies, making sure that the product is free of these things is a wise idea: sugar, salt, wheat, dairy, yeast, preservatives, or artificial colors. Also, if you decide to take some sort of herbal product, find out how much of the active ingredients are actually in the product and whether the company can guarantee you that the herbs are organic and free of pesticides. You don't want to be poisoning yourself on a daily basis with the very thing you are taking to improve your health. Also, check with your medical provider to make sure there are no interactions with other medications or supplements you are taking. Most supplements will need to be stopped prior to any surgical procedure. Just like prescriptive medications, caution must be used with over-the-counter supplements too.

If your budget is limited, you must start somewhere. If you have chosen BHRT, you may need to budget for compounded bioidentical hormones if your insurance plan does not pay for them. Many times, however, the cost of a month's supply of a compounded hormone can be comparable to a co-pay for a trade name product. So don't fret over the price of hormones. They are well worth the trade off since a compounding pharmacy can customize a hormone for each individual person. Being able to titrate dosings in smaller increments than pharmaceuticals ensures that each person is receiving the correct amount of the hormone for his or her specific need(s).

A full-spectrum vitamin that is highly absorbable is a good place to start when it comes to nutritional supplements. That way you can at least be assured that you are getting all of your essential nutrients on a daily basis. I believe that one mistake many women commonly make is taking too much of one or a few nutrients. A good balance of *all* is required by the body. For instance, you may be on a B-complex, omega 3s, calcium, and CoQ10. Those are all well and good, but what about vitamin A, vitamin D, magnesium, copper, zinc, and boron? These are just a few examples of a whole host of other nutrients and trace minerals in which women tend to be deficient. Buying three to four different bottles of a single nutrient can cost anywhere from $20 to $30-plus for each, which can add up quickly to hundreds of dollars each month. Purchasing a quality, highly absorbable, full-spectrum vitamin may cost anywhere from $60 to $150, but will contain *all* of the daily essential nutrients. If some sort of testing then reveals you are low on certain vitamins or minerals, then you can supplement or add to your regimen from there. The idea is that if you are taking a high-quality multi-vitamin and mineral complex, you will most likely get your money's worth and benefit more in the long run. If you want to go the food route, organic fruits and vegetables or a high-quality superfood-type supplement can supply an array of nutrients that will deliver a wide variety of naturally occurring vitamins and minerals, filling in where your diet is lacking. Often these are costly too but may be less than vitamin packages. Remember to take a digestive enzyme with your superfood supplements as most enzymes are destroyed in the manufacturing process.

As you read in the chapter on the intestinal system, I am a stickler for gut health! I am a big fan of probiotics and digestive enzymes. These along with a quality multi-vitamin supplement are three of what I call *essentials* for women of all ages.

Again, include all or some of these in your food budget, medical spending account, or into whatever funds you can distribute these *necessities*. If it looks impossible to do so, cut a few dinners out or find something else in your budget that you are willing to eliminate. When you indeed comprehend the significance and begin to see the advantages of such practices, you will be much more willing to continue to make your health and wellness a priority with your funds. I always remind my clients that the lifestyle changes they are willing to make for the better in their forties and fifties will greatly determine the quality of life they will have in the their sixties, seventies, and beyond. Remember, again, I am talking about prevention. It is far better to prevent disease than to wait until it takes hold and then try and conquer it.

As a Christian provider, I see education as a big part of my responsibility for both physical and moral health principles for living. Individuals need to be taught that drugs do not cure diseases. It is

Discipline is the bridge between
goals and accomplishment.

—John Rohn

absolutely true that they can afford us symptom relief and recovery may come for a period of time as the result of their use and in spite of the poisons they introduce into our systems. This is secondary to this amazing and incredible human creation that God developed. He knew that we would need a system that could compensate for the mistakes we create in our environment. However, the toxins that are introduced and remain in our system for extended periods of time do harm and manifest their effects at a later date.

Again, I believe that too little attention is given to the *prevention* of disease. It is not that I am against research. I believe God and science to be friends and that He reveals Himself to us in our pursuit of science. Who knows what God may reveal and continue to reveal to our scientists in the future? I emphatically support science and research. But think about it—the majority of research is usually conducted and paid for by pharmaceutical companies that are once again looking for a drug, usually toxic substances, that will decrease a symptom, not necessarily cure a disease. Because of this, I think many times they are looking in the wrong place for answers. God has provided us with many natural resources for healing and prevention of disease. I believe we should search for them and use them. I'd like to reiterate that it is far better to prevent a disease than to treat it when the disease is contracted. We have many "Walk-for-the-Cure" fundraisers. What about a "Walk-for-Prevention?" That never happens because the bottom line is the almighty dollar. Few are willing to spend much or any money to promote prevention of disease because it does not bring in the dollars like drugs and pharmaceuticals do.

One would think that the insurance companies would want to allow preventative measures for their clients (it would certainly save them millions in the future), but even that industry has not caught on to the incredible benefits and savings for their companies when preventative health care is pursued. How unfortunate. Therefore, we have to take the responsibility into our own hands, buckle down, and just do it ourselves. Jordon Rubin, NMD, CNC, says that the insurance industry is largely dependent on statistics. The average life span and principal causes of premature death are continuously studied. Yet no statistician is willing to really spell out the paramount cause of death among the human race, and that is ignorance.[1] Whoa, that hurts! If I am going to die, let it be secondary to natural causes and God's will in my life, not because I am unwilling to take the time to read, learn, discern for myself, and take appropriate action. The fact that you are reading this book is solid evidence that you are seeking and on that learning path. Blessings to you on that pursuit.

Self-control is certainly a health principle that can pay big benefits. We have lost self-control in a number of areas of our lives. Man's loss of self-control has destroyed more than our health. The lack of self-control is, again, another example of why our economy is failing. We can't wait! Anything that our will desires, it seems we must have it and have it now. Our bodies and our minds must be brought into subjection. And it is impossible to do this on our own. The only way is to place ourselves under the control of God. By practicing the principle of self-discipline, and in some cases self-denial, God can help us be successful in all areas of our lives. Paul wrote in 1 Corinthians 9:27, "I discipline my body like an athlete training it to do what it should. Otherwise, after preaching to others I myself might be disqualified" (NLT). We need the divine power to make lifestyle changes in the way of spending habits and health habits that are right. With Christ's help we can be "a living sacrifice, holy and without blemish, well pleasing to God" (Rom. 12:1).

Don't tell me where your priorities are. Show me where you spend your money and I'll tell you what they are.

—James W. Frick

Chapter 10

❧

Your Story, My Story

What is your story? Some of you reading this book have good health. Nothing really bad in the way of health concerns has ever crossed your path. For those of you in that situation, I say, "Praise God!" In matters related to a health crisis, I have always said to my children, "Just wait, because it is not if but when." Somewhere in your life, it *will* come—if not to yourself, then maybe to a very close friend, family member, or relative. The reality of this world is that we must learn to number our days. Psalm 90:10, 12 says, "The length of our days is seventy years-or eighty, if we have the strength; yet their span is but trouble and sorrow, for they quickly pass, and we fly away ... teach us to number our days aright, that we may gain a heart of wisdom" (NIV). We must remember that this is not our home and eventually we are all destined to meet eternity. Are you ready?

Many of you understand this more thoroughly because you have not had such smooth sailing along the way. You may have endured all kinds of physical or emotional situations. Daily life has become a struggle. Although this book offers some suggestions, I have no clear advice or answers to those of you in that particular kind of situation. I do know, though, that there are many women just like you facing similar problems and their offering help in the way of a listening ear can be comforting. I envision there is nothing more disturbing than optimistic words belted from someone who has never walked in your shoes. However, refreshment can come from simple and quiet words of those whose lives have seen and experienced troubled times similar to yours. Your words of encouragement also can be a treasure to others like you. Sometimes God shines His strength and light best through our brokenness.

At this writing, I personally have pretty good health. Yes, I have a few occasional minor aches and pains here and there but nothing major. I am very thankful to God every day for that blessing. However, I am sixty years old and have lived through some challenging times and events. My childhood was good, but as I grew to be a teenager, there were some emotional pangs. I have had four surgeries, two major. I have had four pregnancies, three deliveries, and one miscarriage. I have lived through both the joys and heartaches of raising three children and now am watching eight grandchildren grow. I watched my father face the complications of diabetes, heart disease, limb amputation, lung cancer, brain cancer, and finally death. I saw the incredible sufferings as my mother fought chronic migraine headaches, rheumatoid arthritis, lupus, heart disease, osteoporosis, kidney and lung disease, a major stroke, and eventually death. These were terribly heartbreaking on all accounts.

I have seen and continue to experience emotional pains with my clients, family, and friends over health issues, marriage problems, alcoholism, drug abuse, suicide, loss of family members, and the list goes on and on. None of these have been or are pleasant things to face or endure. How I have prayed and yearned for *all* that this life wouldn't hold such trials and tribulations. But looking back, I cannot think of one situation where Christ has not taught me an eternal lesson or given me some amount of wisdom to share with those around me. So for His glory, I thank Him for those trials and tribulations. For "who shall separate us from the love of Christ? Shall trouble or hardship? No, in all these things we are more than conquerors through Him who loved us" (Rom. 5:35–37). I know that most of you have been given that same gift from your life experiences and that they can and will be used by God too. We need to be able to laugh together, cry together, listen to each other, and learn from one another. These are gifts we can give that need no particular training or talent. These are the gifts that we can offer each other no matter what our personal situations may be. These are the gifts that I know personally come back to us threefold and in ways we can never imagine. I encourage you to use your particular gifts and use them frequently and wisely.

The power of love to change bodies is legendary, built into folklore, common sense, and everyday experience. Love moves the flesh, it pushes matter around. Throughout history, "tender loving care" has uniformly been recognized as a valuable element in healing.

—Larry Dossey

I understand that many people think if they do not have their health, they have nothing. Well, I am certainly the first to say and admit that health is right up there at the top of my list in terms of importance. Hopefully I have shared some very important information in this book that will help get you on the right path to health and keeping your body strong. However, I personally believe if you don't have Jesus, *then* you don't have *anything*! That to me is the most important thing in *this* life! Hopefully the same is true for you, too. I believe that we must come to the place in our spiritual journey that Christ is first and foremost *all* that we need. We must be willing at any point to let go of anything God allows to be taken away, health included. Our own personal security for now and eternity will always lie in our Savior, but while in the here and now, we must look beyond the circumstances of life and find some good purpose for which they can be used. There will always be situations that are dark to our understanding, but we must come to the place where there is total and complete trust that out of it all God will use it for the higher purpose. Again, that is the gift!

I feel very strongly that for this season of my life God has given me a particular mission and gift to use—serving, teaching, and ministering to you women in the areas of wellness and prevention of disease. It is my yearning that God will continue to accomplish in me this specific purpose in whatever ways He may choose. I also pray that this book has in some way illuminated my deep passion for both your spiritual and physical well-being. Furthermore, I hope I have been able to inspire you with my strong convictions about how you should view and take care of your body, mind, and spirit. Blessings on that pursuit!

God sovereignly and lovingly orchestrates all of time and eternity. He is coordinating every detail of His plan for us so that it interacts perfectly with every detail of the plans for other people, weaving them together like a holy tapestry.

—Bob Coy
Dreamality

My Prayer for You

Lord, I pray that You will hold each woman reading this book close. I pray that it would be her heart's desire to know You better and that she will become so close to You that the path(s) she chooses to take will be directly in line with Your eternal will for her.

Amen

**Note: Please, don't forget to utilize the appendices for your benefit.

References

Chapter 1 (Hormones)

1. Wilson, James L., ND, DC, PhD, *Adrenal Fatigue: The 21ˢᵗ Century Stress Syndrome.* (Petaluma, CA: Smart Publications, 2001), 219–20.
2. Schwarzbein, Diana, MD, *The Schwarzbein Principle II: The Transition.* (Deerfield Beach, FL: Health Communications, Inc., 2002), 24–25.
3. Lam, Michael, MD, *Estrogen Dominance.* Retrieved April 13, 2011, from http://www.drlam.com/articles/Estrogen_Dominance.asp.
4. Hotze, Steven F., MD, *Hormones, Health, and Happiness: A Natural Medical Formula for Rediscovering Youth with Bioidentical Hormones.* (New York: Warner Wellness, 2005), 99.
5. Ibid., 99–100.
6. Ibid,. 100.
7. Null, Gary, *Women's Health Solutions.* (New York: Seven Stories Press, 2002), 122–23.
8. Hotze, *Hormones, Health, and Happiness*, 100.
9. Tuggle, Alex, L.Ac. *Estrogen Dominance Symptoms.* Retrieved August 26, 2010 from http://www.holistic-back-relief.com/estrogen-dominance-symptoms.html.
10. Hotze, *Hormones, Health, and Happiness*, 101–3.
11. Null, *Women's Health Solutions*, 451.
12. Burnett, Reddi. *Influence of estrogen and progesterone on matrix-induced endochondral bone Formation,* Calcif Tissue Int. 1983,Jul; 35(4-5); 609–14. PMID: 6616325 [PubMed—indexed for MEDLINE].
13. Hotze, *Hormones, Health, and Happiness*, 105.
14. Lee, John R., MD, Zava, David, PhD, and Hopkins, Virginia, *What Your Doctor May Not Tell You About Breast Cancer: How Hormone Balance Can Help Save Your Life. (New York:* Warner Wellness, 2003), 166.
15. Hotze, *Hormones, Health, and Happiness*, 105.

16. Iasif. *Effects of protracted administration of estriol on the lower genito urinary tract in postmenopausal women,* Department of Obstetrics and Gynecology, University of Lund, Sweden; Arch Gynecololgy and Obstetrics. 1992; 251(3): 115–20. PMID: 1605676 [PubMed—indexed for MEDLINE].

17. Raz, Stamum. *A controlled trial of intravaginal estriol in postmenopausal women with recurrent urinary tract infections.* Infectious Disease Unit, Central Emek Hospital, Afula, Israel. N. Engi J Med, 1993, Sept 9; 329(11); 753–6. www.contet.nejm.org.

18. Conley, Edward, MD, *Safe Estrogen: Reduce Your Breast Cancer Risk By 90%. (Flint, MI:* Vitality Press, Inc., 2003), 18.

19. Cheng, Maria (2010). *Up to a Third of Breast Cancers Could Be Avoided,* Retrieved March 25, 2010, from http://news.yahoo.com/s/ap/20100325/ap_on_he_me/eu_med_avoiding_breast_cancer.

20. Conley, *Safe Estrogen,* 52.

21. Ibid., 13.

22. Lee, Zava, Hopkins, *What Your Doctor May Not Tell You about Breast Cancer,* 193.

23. Sellers, Mink, Cerhan, Zheng, Anderson, Kushi, Folsom. *The role of hormone replacement therapy in the risk for breast cancer and total mortality in women with a family history of breast cancer,* Division of epidemiology, University of Minnesota, Minneapolis; ACP J Club. 1998 May–Jun; 128(3):74: PMID: 9412302 [PubMed—indexed for MEDLINE].

24. Natrajan, Soumakis, Gambrell Jr. *Estrogen replacement therapy in women with previous breast cancer,* Department of Physiology, Medical College of Georgia, Georgia; Am J Obstetrics and Gynecology 1999 Aug; 181(2):288–95. PMID: 10454671 [PubMed—indexed for MEDLINE].

25. Conley, *Safe Estrogen,* 102.

26. Lee, John R., M.D. *John R. Lee's Three Rules for Hormone Replacement Therapy.* Retrieved April 13, 2011, from http://www.johnleemd.com/store/news_bhrt.html.

27. Hotze, *Hormones, Health, and Happiness,* 5–6.

28. Sherwin. *Can Estrogen Keep You Smart? Evidence from a Clinical Studies,* Department of Psychology, McGill University, Montreal, Que.: Journal of Psychiatry Neuroscience 1999, September; 24(4): 315–21. PMID: 10516798 [PubMed—indexed for MEDLINE].

29. Smith, Pamela Wartian, MD, *HRT: The Answers,* Traverse City, MI: Healthy Living Books, Inc., 2003), 78.

30. Endo Resolve (2010). *Estrogen Foods and the Diet for Endometriosis—Why There is Confusion*. Retrieved September 1, 2010, from http://www.endo-resolved.com.diet_phytoestrogens.html.

31. Ibid.

32. Ibid.

33. Lininger, S., Gaby, A., et. al, *The Natural Pharmacy*, Rocklin, CA: Healthnotes, Inc., 1999), 470.

Chapter 2 (Heart Health and Beyond)

1. Centers for Disease Control and Prevention (February 24, 2011). *Heart Disease is the Number One Cause of Death*, Retrieved February 24, 2011, from http://www.cdc.gov/features/heartmonth.

2. Hopel, Ann M., Editor, "Women's Health in the U.S.," *Clinical Reviews*, February 2011, Vol. 21, No. 2, pages 1, 17, 28.

3. Streib, Lauren. *World's Fattest Countries*. Retrieved March 16, 2011, from http://www.forbes.com/2007/02/07/worlds-fattest-countries-forbeslife-cx_1s_0208worldfat.

4. Northrup, Christiane, MD, *Women's Bodies, Women's Wisdom*. (New York: Bantam Books, 1998), 563.

5. Hotze, *Hormones, Health, and Happiness*, 204–5.

6. Louet, J., LeMay C., and Mauvais-Jarvis, F., *Antidiabetic Actions of Estrogen: Insight from human and Genetic Mouse Models*, Current Artherosclerosis Reports, Volume 6, Number 3, 180–5 DOI:10,1007/s11883-004-0030- 9. Retrieved February 24, 2011, from http://www.springerlink.com/Content/j792457607690277/.

7. *Hormonally Challenged*, Retrieved May 4, 2011, from http://blog.seattleepi.com/hormonallychallenged/2008/05/15/cholesterol-abd-hormones/.

8. Spectracell Laboratories (2011). *Do Cholesterol Numbers Assess Cardiovascular Risk?* Retrieved July 18, 2011 from http://sss.spectracell.com.lpp/.

9. Schwartzbein, Diana, MD, *The Schwarzbein Principle II*, 102.

10. Hotze, *Hormones, Health, and Happiness*, 137.

11. Ibid, 138.

12. Schwartzbein, *The Schwarzbein Principle II*, 101.

13. *High Blood Pressure: Test and Diagnoisis*. Retrieved March 28, 2011, from http://www.mayoclinic.com/health/high-blood-pressure/DS00100/DSECTION=tests-and-diagnosis.

14. Cummings, Benjamin. *Factors that Affect Blood Pressure.* Retrieved May 12, 2011 from www.aw- bc.com/info/ip/.

15. Sheps, Sheldon G., MD, *High Blood Pressure: What is Pulse Pressure? How Important is Pulse Pressure to Your Overall Health?* Retrieved March 28, 2011, from http://www.mayoclinic.com/health/pulse-pressure/AN00968.

16. Null, Gary, *Women's Health Solutions.* (New York: Seven Stories Press, 2002), 287–8.

17. Wise Pharmacy, *The Mortar and Pestle* (April 2010). *Is Transdermal Estradiol + Progesterone the Preferred Postmenopausal HRT? Brit Med J 1986; 290:34.*

18. Hotze, 220.

19. Smith, *HRT: The Answers*, 70.

20. Ibid, 71.

21. Weil, Andrew (2002), February. *Self-Healing, Creating Health for Your Body and mind*, (February, 2002). New Risk Factors for Heart Disease, 4.

22. Ibid, 4.

23. Brouqui et al. 1994; Devaux et al. 1997; DeKeyser et al. 1998. *Aging and Inflammation*, Retrieved May 4, 2011, from http://www.lef.org/protocals/prtcl-146.shtml.

24. Smith, 73.

25. Decensi A, Omodei U, Robertson C, Bonnani B, Guerrieri-Gonzaga A, Ramazzotto F, Johansson H, Mora S, Sandri MT, Cazzaniga M, Franchi M, Pecorelli S. *Effect of Transdermal Estradiol and Oral Conjugated Estrogen on C-Reactive Protein in Retinoid-Placebo Trial in Healthy Women.* Retrieved June 27, 2011 from http://www.ncbI.nlm.nih.gov/pubmed/12208797.

26. Information for the Public: *Questions and Answers About Estrogen-Plus-Progestin Hormone Therapy.* Retrieved July 21, 2011 from http://nhlbi.nih.gov/health/women/q_a.htm.

27. Smith, 72.

28. Jigsaw Health. *Thick Blood: Common Causes.* Retrieved March 28, 2011 from http://www.jigsawhealth.com/resources/thickk-blood-causes.

29. Smith, 71.

30. *Check Iron Levels Postmenopause To Determine Need for Supplements.* Medical Edge Newspaper Column, October 10, 2008. Retrieved March 28, 2011, from http://www.mayoclinic.org/medical-edge-newspaper-2008/oct-10b.html.

31. Graveline, Duane, MD. *Post Menopausal Iron Supplementation—Caution!* Retrieved March 28, 2011, from http://www.spacedoc.net/post_menopausal_iron_supplementation.

32. Am, J. Serum *Ferritin and bone marrow biopsy iron stores. 11. Correlation with low serum iron and Fe/TIBC Ratio less than 15%.* U.S. National Library of Medicine. 1980 Oct; 74(4);461–4. PMID:7424828 [PubMed—Indexed for MEDLINE].

33. Dubey, Gillespie, Jackson, Keller. *17Beta-Estraiol, its metabolites, and progesterone inhibit cardiac fibroblast growth*, Department of Medicine, University of Pittsburgh Medical Center, PA; hypertension. 1998 Jan, 31 (1 Pt 2): 522-B: PMID:9453356 [PubMed—indexed for MEDLINE].

34. Holtorf, Kent MD. *The Bioidentical Hormone Debate: Are Bioidentical Hormones Safer or More Efficacious than Commonly Used Synthetic Version in Hormone Replacement Therapy?* Postgraduate Medicine, Volume 121, Issue I, January 2009, ISSN-0032-5481, e-ISSN-1941-9260.

Chapter 3 (Hypothyroid)

1. Brownstein, David, *Overcoming Thyroid Disorders*, Second Edition. West Bloomfield, MI: Medical Alternatives Press, 2002), 35.

2. Ibid.

3. Ibid, 43.

4. Hotze, *Hormones, Health, and Happiness*, 68.

5. Brownstein, 34.

6. Ibid., 45.

7. Hotze, 70.

8. Schwarzbein, *The Schwarzbein Principle II* , 45.

9. Hotze, 69–70.

10. Browstein, 110.

11. Hotze, 70.

12. Ibid., 71.

13. Brownstein, 252.

14. Lycos Retriever. *Iodine: Iodine Deficiency Disorders.* Retrieved May 4, 2011, from http://www.lycos.com/info/iodine--iodine-deficiency-disorders.html.

15. Ibid, Brownstein, page 84.

16. Sarver, Robert. *Iodine Deficiency* (Copyright 2005). Retrieved May 4, 2011, from http://www.vitamincfoundation.org/iodine.htm.

17. Brownstein, 291.

Chapter 4 (Digestion)

1. Rubin, Jordan S., NMD, CNC., *Patient Heal Thyself*, Topanga, CA: Freedom Press, 2003), 47.
2. Fuller, DicQie, PhD, DSc, *The Healing Power of Enzymes, How Enzyme Supplements Can Turn Your Life Around.* (New York: Forbes Custom Publishing, 2002), 13–14.
3. Ibid., 3.
4. Ibid., 171.
5. Ibid., 11.
6. Ibid., 183–4.
7. Kafka, Kathy. *Intestinal Parasites.* Retrieved June 28, 2010, from http://www.articlebase.com/diseases-and-conditions-articles/intestinal-parasites-751540.h.
8. Rubin, 67–68.
9. Ibid., 50.

Chapter 5 (Adrenals)

1. Wilson, 3.
2. Ibid., 8.
3. Ibid., 9.
4. Ibid., 219.
5. Ibid., 220–1.

Chapter 6 (Toxicity)

1. Environmental Resources Center. (2003, July). *The True Cost of Petroleum* (Electronic Version), 1–2.
2. Crinnion, Walter, M.D. *Our Toxic Enviornment.* Retrieved March 3, 2011, from http://www.crinnionmedical.com/Crinnion_medical/Environment _Medicine.html.
3. Ibid, Crinnion.
4. Hanshew, Lyn, MD, *ACZ and Radiation.* Retrieved March 31, 2011, from http://us.mc1129.mail.yahoo.com/mc/showMessage?sMid=5&filter By=&.rand=13223470.
5. *Understanding the Lymphatic System.* Retrieved March 3, 2011 from http://www.lymphomation.org/lymphatic.htm.
6. Standley, Loretta J., MD *The Lymphatic System.* Retrieved March 3, 2011 from http://drstandley.com/bodysystems_lymphatic.shtml.

7. Environmental Resources Center.

8. Ibid..

9. *Heavy Metal Toxicity: Mercury Detoxification*. Retrieved March 17, 2010, from http://tuberose.com/heavy_ Metal_toxicity.html.

10. Ibid.

11. Collin, Jonsthan, M.D. (2004, July 14). *EDTA Chelation Therapy*. Retrieved July 12, 2010, from http://www.townsendletter.com/Chelation/chelation.jc.c.htm

12. Crinnion.

Chapter 7 (Yeast)

1. The Yeast Among Us. *The Ground-breaking Work of Dr. Orian Truss And Other Pioneers*. Retrieved August 16, 2011, from http://www.drdemarco.com/charge/pg74/htm.

2. *Candida—New Theories, New Cures*, Retrieved July 7, 2010, from http://wddty.com/candida_1.hhtml.

3. Ibid.

4. Ibid.

5. One Sweet Nation. Available in U.S. News and World Report, March 28, 2005. Retrieved July 12, 2010 from http://health.usnews.com/usnews/health/articles/050328/28sugar.b.htm.

6. CSPI Newsroom (2000). *Sugar Intake Hit All Time High in 1999: Government Urged to Recommend Sugar Limits*. Retrieved July 12, 2010, from http://www.cspinet.org/new/sugar_limit.html.

7. Amber Waves (2005). U.S. Food Consumption up 16 Percent Since 1970, Retrieved July 12, 2010, from http://www.ers.esda.gov/amberwaves/november05/findings/USfoodconsumption.htm.

8. One Sweet Nation.

9. *American Drowning in Sugar: Experts Call for Food Labels to Disclose Added Sugars (1999)*. Retrieved July 12, 2010, from http://www.cspinet.org/net/sugar.html.

10. Ibid, CSPI Newsroom.

11. Bandyopadhyay, A, Ghoshal, S, Mukherjee, A. *Genotoxicity Testing of Low Calorie Sweetners: Aspartame, Acesulfame-k and Saccharin*, 2008, Vol 31, No. 4, p. 447–57. Retrieved April 12, 2011 from http://informahealthcare.com/doi/abs.10.1080.01480540802390270.

12. Filippini M., Maslero G., Moschetti K., (2005*). Socioeconomic determinants of regional differences in outpatient Antibiotic consumption: Evidence from Switzerland*, Retrieved July 12, 2010 from www.sciencedirect.com.

13. Ibid.

14. Null, 247.

15. Trudeau, Kevin, *Natural Cures They Don't Want You to Know About*, Hinsdale, IL: Alliance Publishing Group, Inc., 2004), 93.

16. Null, 247.

17. Ferlise M. *The Demand for Prescription Drugs: An Analysis of the United States.* The College of New Jersey 2002; 1–4.

18. NJ.com (2010, May 19). *Medco Report Shows Spending Increase on Drugs for Kids.* Retrieved July 12, 2010, from http://www.nj.com/business/index.ssf/2010/05/Medco_report_shows_spending_in.html.

19. Lipski, Elizabeth, PhD., CCN. *Digestive Wellness, Third Edition. (Colombus, OH:* McGraw Hill, 2005), 69.

20. Ibid, Page 69.

21. *Making the Yeast Connection*, Retrieved April 12, 2011 from http://www.wddty.com/making- the-yeast-connection.html.

22. Sellman, Sherrill, ND**,** *The Total Body Detox Solution,* Retrieved August 22, 2011, from http://www.resultsrna.com.

23. Enzyme Stuff, the wonderful world of enzymes, *Enzymes for Fighting Yeast*, Retrieved August 16, 2001, from httP:// www.enzymestuff.com/conditionyeast.htm.

24. Crook, William G., MD, *The Yeast Connection Handbook. (Jackson, TN:* Women's Health Connection, Inc., 2000), 129–30.

25. Ibid., 130.

26. Ibid., 130–1.

27. Ibid., 132.

28. Ibid., 132–3.

Chapter 8 (PMRT)

1. Carmichael, Joel P., DC, DACBSP, *Magnetic Resonance Stimulation, Using the Field to Maximize Your Health*, NAAcEM, Edition I, 2009, 16.

2. Thuile, Christian, MD. *Practice of Magnetic Field Therapy,* Published by the International Association of Energy Medicine (IGEM), English Edition, 2000, 13.

3. Carmichael, 41.

4. Ibid., 45.

5. Becker, Robert O. *Electromagnetic Radiation Safety.* Retrieved July 13, 2011 from http://emr- safety.blogspot.com/2008/05/robert-o-becker-1923-2008.html.
6. Thuile, 24.
7. Ibid., 6.
8. Ibid., 7.
9. *Information, Magentic Resonance Stimulation.* Brochure published by the National Academy of Energy Medicine (NA AcEM).

Chapter 9 (Money and Health Principles)

1. Rubin, Jordan S., NMD, CNC, *Patient Heal Thyself.* (Topanga, CA: Freedom Press, 2003), 66.

Appendix I

&

Judy's Favorite Supplements

Please Note: I am not dedicated to one particular line of products. The supplement industry is huge, and every company is out to make its bucks. I just do my research and choose products I have clinically or personally experienced to be the best products that have sound research behind them, come from reputable companies, and last but not least give the best performance (stood the test of time) in the area for which that particular product is indicated. Some of the products may be from a MLM company, and others may not. In my brief summary of each product, I explain why I chose that particular product or brand over another. This is not to say that you cannot find other products or brands out there that may be just as good as the ones I have chosen. Also, I am not claiming that any of these products will cure any disease.

1. Multi-Vitamins:

Lifepak Nano: This is my personal vitamin. It is what I believe to be one of the most comprehensive vitamins on the market today. It not only contains all of the necessary vitamins and minerals, but it also contains high-powered antioxidants and phytonutrients, CoQ10, mercury-free krill oil, and more. Many of these nutrients, like the omega 3s, specific vitamins, carotenoids, and CoQ10, are manufactured with nanotechnology to increase absorption and are guaranteed to increase your skin carotenoid score. Although this vitamin package is rather expensive, I have found that I actually save money because everything that should be in a multi-vitamin and more is in this package ($122/box of sixty packets, recommended two packets per day). **

StarPac: This is another great, high-quality vitamin package. I chose this as a second multi-vitamin option because it was created with a micellization process that also helps the vitamins break down easily in the stomach, therefore increasing absorption. It is in a tablet form versus capsules, so vegans prefer this choice, as well as anyone else wanting a high-quality, reasonably priced multi-vitamin. This vitamin includes all the essential vitamins and minerals, omega 3 and 6 essential fatty acids, gamma linolenic and linoleic acids, phytonutrients, and a specially selected enzyme complex with thirty naturally occurring enzymes to aid in the digestion process ($49/thirty packets).**

2. Probiotics:

ProFlora Concentrate: A probiotic formulation containing one billion flora in a seamless caplet designed by the Japanese to withstand the acids of the stomach. This caplet does not break down until it gets into the intestines and then begins to deposit the flora along the intestines and colon where they belong. ProFlora Concentrate does not have to be refrigerated, making it ideal for travel too. My personal favorite for probiotic maintenance ($25/thirty count, $60/ninety count).**

Probiotic Pearls Advantage: The same formulation as above, but contains five billion flora in a seamless caplet. I recommend this probiotic formulation during cold and flu season or to establish flora colonies in the intestines if one has not taken probiotics in the past or is trying to increase the immune system quickly ($60/sixty count).**

3. Detoxes:

VelociTea, also known as Holy Tea: This medicinal tea is an herbal preparation that first works in the colon cleansing the intestines from worms and parasites. Once the intestines are cleansed, it begins cleansing toxins from the liver and then the blood and other tissues. It helps with maintaining weight as well as bowel function and more. This tea may be used as part of a weight-loss program. It can be consumed hot or cold, mixed with juice, or added to your favorite beverage. The tea is not bitter and is easily tolerated. You can buy online wholesale at: http://www.wholewellnessclub.net/judyponsford ($40/four packages).**

Advanced Cellular Silver (ACS): ACS is a ribosomal RNA intra-oral spray that is independently proven to be the most powerful anti-microbial available. It kills 99.9999 percent of MRSA (Methicillin-resistant staphylococcus aureus) and Candida in less than three minutes. It provides powerful immune system support. It is antifungal, antiviral, and bacteriacidal. I use this clinically for a natural bacterial, viral, and yeast cleanse. It is very safe and the spray formula, is easily tolerated and more effective than any natural detox that goes through the digestive system. It also comes in a SuperShot formula for acute illnesses, such as flu or colds ($50/four-ounce bottle, SuperShot $30).** You may read more about this and other RNA products listed below at: http://www.resultsrna.com. Sold only by providers.**

4. Chelation:

Advanced Cellular Zeolite (ACZ): ACZ is a ribosomal RNA intra-oral spray that eliminates heavy metals, neurotoxins, radioactive isotopes, and free radicals. It is proven to increase urinary output of mercury, lead, and other heavy metals by 300 percent. The nano-sized zeolite crystals provide a greater surface area detox. This product also balances pH levels and supports a healthy immune system ($65/four-ounce bottle).** The Total Body Detox Kit which contains both the four-ounce Advanced Cellular Silver and Zeolite is $100.** To check for neurotoxins, go to: http://www.chronicneurotoxins.com and take the $15 test created by Dr. Shoemaker. Sold only by providers.

Peak Enzymes "Without": These systemic/metabolic enzymes are some of the most powerful on the market today. These particular enzymes mainly contain protease, serrapeptase, and nattokinase. Protease will digest any protein particles that do not belong in the blood stream that may be causing allergic reactions. Serrapeptase is taken from the silk worm and digests nonliving particles. In the blood, it will digest everything that is not supposed to be there, from uric acid crystals to plaque in the arteries. Nattokinase resembles the plasmin and helps dissolve fibrin, keeping the blood running smoothly and making it less sticky. This product also helps reduce inflammation in the body, reduce cholesterol, balance blood sugars, and cleanse plaque from the arteries ($60/ninety count).** You may read more information about this product or purchase wholesale at: http://www.wholewellnessclub.net/judyponsford.

5. Superfoods/Greenfoods:

SalbaRx: Salba seeds are an antiaging superfood and a great gluten replacement that can be added to almost any food. It is relatively tasteless, not grainy or chalky, with zero caffeine. It contains high levels of Omega 3 fatty acids, vegetable protein, fiber, calcium, magnesium, vitamin C, plus twenty-four other nutrients. It may help to rebuild cells, stabilize blood sugars, reduce blood pressure, reduce cholesterol, give antioxidant protection, flush out toxins, regulate bowels, stabilize sleep pattern, boost energy, and control weight. Unlike regular salba seeds, the Rx formula contains maca root, which helps to balance hormones. Much more nutritious than flax seed ($45/twenty ounces).**

Sun Chlorella: This is the best and only pulverized chlorella on the market today. The patented pulverization process breaks down chlorella's tough outer cell wall, which ensures maximum bioavailability, digestion, and assimilation of the chlorella. Sun Chlorella "A" is the only chlorella to contain 95 percent pulverized cell wall without using heat or chemicals. It contains the nutritionally superior species of *Chlorella paranoids* ($30/bag of 120 count or a box of five bags for $130).**

Caldera Greens: These greens come from a caldera. This is a volcanic crater much like Yellowstone National Park. The volcanic soil on this caldera is extremely rich in minerals and fulvic acid. Fulvic acid is nature's very best natural electrolyte. The farm is fully integrated, meaning the food is grown, harvested, processed, and packaged on the grounds. Within five hours of harvest, all of the crops are juiced and dried at the most noninvasive, low temperature of 88°F. This food is truly alive! All of the enzymes and soil-based organisms are intact. Caldera greens supply all nutrients the human body needs. It is alkalizing, helps repair DNA, acts as free radical scavengers, helps improve skin health, stimulates weight loss, and more. It comes in powdered form as well as capsules for easy and convenient consumption. It can be purchased at: http://www.wholewellnessclub.net/judyponsford ($46/220 gms or 300 caps).**

6. Digestive Enzymes:

Peak Enzymes "With": This is a reasonably priced and good-quality full-spectrum enzyme that aids digestion. This is my personal daily enzyme. You may read more information about these enzymes and purchase wholesale at: http://wholewellnessclub.net /judyponsford ($28/ninety count).**

Digestive Enzymes Ultra: This is another one of my favorite full-spectrum enzymes from Pure Encapsulations. It is high in both protease and amylase making is a good choice for those who have protease and/or amylase deficiencies ($25/ninety count).**

Lipase Concentrate H-P: This particular enzyme by Integrative Therapeutics, Inc., is often used in addition to a full-spectrum digestive enzyme. Lipase can benefit someone who has had their gallbladder removed, has tested lipase deficient, or struggles with weight gain or obesity.

7. Brain Function:

Neuro Care: This was created by ResultsRNA, the same company that manufactures the ACS and ACZ detox products recommended above. It is an intra-oral spray that increases brain function. If you are having trouble with your words or thought process, this may be the answer to better brain function ($35/two-ounce bottle).** This is another one of my personal favorites. **

8. Inflammation:

Zyphlamend: This is a natural antiinflammatory product by New Chapter. I highly recommend this product to anyone who has any type of arthritic condition or whose C-reactive protein levels are above 1.0 mg/L ($32.95–$34.95/sixty count).**

wwc pH Control: This product includes glutathione, one of the most potent antioxidants, as well as other vitamins and minerals. Remember, the more alkaline you are, the less disease you will have. This product is tops in this category since it is inhaled and is distributed throughout the body via the lungs ($58/four-ounce bottle).** May be purchased online at: http://www. wholewellnessclub.net/judyponsford.

Advanced Cellular Glutathione (ACG): This is a ribosomal intra-oral spray from the same company that produces ACS and ACZ. Glutathione is the most critical intracellular antioxidant. Glutathione regulates all other antioxidants while preventing damage to important cellular components caused by free radicals and peroxides. Getting glutathione into the system has been difficult in the past, but with this intra-oral spray, instant bioavailability to the system is now possible. If you need a good antioxidant or want to reduce inflammation in the system, this is a superior product ($45/two-ounce bottle).**

9. All in One Supplement

Natraburst: This is one of those supplements for people who hate to take tablets or capsules. It has a wide range of nutrients including superfoods, greenfoods, antioxidants, amino acids, protein, fiber, natural vitamins and minerals, as well as probiotics and digestive enzymes. Contains no gluten, MSG, soy, or artificial flavors or sweeteners. A great all around supplement. Makes a great morning shake. This is part of my daily breakfast ($69.95/30 scoops). Can be purchased at: http://www.judyponsford.124online.com. Click on the "order retail" link and follow the prompts.

10. Something New

Homeopathic HgH: HgH is natural to the body, just like all your other hormones. Research on life extension in the last forty years has centered around human growth hormone (HgH), a substance that is secreted by the pituitary gland. Like most hormones, it is abundant in the body while young but starts to decline dramatically after eighteen and particularly after the age of thirty. The problem with getting HgH in the past has been the fact that it has only been available in injection form and was very expensive. Even if one could afford the injections, it is most beneficial to multi-inject throughout the day, is invasive, and can have side effects. Other advertised products only "tickle" the pituitary to help it produce more HgH for a while, and then the pituitary gets used to the "tickle" and the products stop working. Also, these products contain no traces of HgH hormone, although these supplement companies often advertise them as HgH products. Now there is a new solution, homeopathic HgH!

Homeopathics are gentle, safe, and very effective, with little chance of side effects compared to the various molecular (injectable) HgH and stacked amino/seretagogue (digestible) HgH products. Medical studies show that small amounts of HgH taken at frequent intervals work better, and that is one of the basic principles of homeopathy. Homeopathic HgH does not interfere with any other supplement or medicine that an individual might be taking … with the exception that sometimes the positive benefits of homeopathic HgH can help one reduce or even come off of other medications. Homeopathic HgH gently encourages the pituitary to release and supplement HgH and balance the body. This is called homeostasis. According to homeopathic principles, the succussion process actually makes the HgH potent, or dynamic, so it is even more bioactive in the body. The homeopathic process energizes any elements that are produced in this manner.

The homeopathic theory of dilution and succussion teaches that molecules can penetrate the cells more easily. This process also causes the HgH to act as a "timed release" agent in the body. Therefore, it doesn't matter when you take the homeopathic version, you still get a very good result and the homeopathic factors continue to work in the body, even when you may forget a dosing or two. It's gentle and completely safe. Try it; you will like it ($55/one ounce—a six-week supply). Advanced formula ($85/one ounce—a six-week supply).**

Below are some of the documented benefits of this product:

- Muscle mass increase and tone without increased exercise

- Reduced fat and cellulite without a change in diet or habits
- Enhanced sexual performance
- Increased cardiac output
- Better kidney function
- Increased HDL (good cholesterol) and decreased LDL (bad cholesterol)
- Faster wound healing
- Regrowth/recolor of hair
- Mood elevation
- Improved sleep
- Balanced hormones
- Regeneration in growth of heart, liver, and kidney
- Increased immune function
- Increase in strength and exercise performance
- Decrease in blood pressure
- Stronger bones
- Younger-looking and thicker skin
- Decrease in wrinkling
- Increase in memory
- Decrease in menopausal symptoms

11. Essential Oils:

Essential Oils: If you have not experienced the health benefits of essential oils, you are missing out! Just like herbs and other natural plant extracts, essential oils are God's *very special* gift to us for health and healing. Essential oils have a bioelectrical frequency several times higher than that of herbs, food, or even the human body. Essential oils can rapidly raise the frequency of the body, making them oxygenating, detoxifying, regenerating, powerful free radical scavengers, and immune defense agents. Essential oils are lipid-soluble and can affect every cell in the body within twenty minutes of use and then be metabolized like any other nutrient. The molecular structure of essential oils is so small that they can quickly penetrate the skin and cell walls; and those containing sesquiterpenes can cross the blood-brain barrier, enabling them to be effective treatments for neurological problems such as Alzheimer's disease, Lou Gehrig's disease, Parkinson's multiple sclerosis, and more. There are specific essential oils or blends of oils beneficial for every physical or emotional ailment. No household should be without some of these oils. One of my favorites is Thieves. No household should be without it. Do your own research, and then try some out at: http://www.youngliving.com. Use Distributor **#1292238**. No membership fee is required to learn about or order products. Click on the "member sign-up" link in the upper right hand corner and follow the prompts. Each oil or oil blend is priced individually.

Adaptogen:

Laminine: Laminine is a form of a natural adaptogen which helps to create a state of balance or normalization of the body - homeostasis. Laminine is my adaptogen of choice. Our bodies contain a cross-shaped molecular structure protein that is encoded into our DNA and is literally considered the *"glue that holds us together!"* This protein's availability diminishes over time and eventually vanishes. The reduction in this protein can cause rapid aging and health-related problems. Miraculously, LifePharm Global Network has created Laminine which acts just like laminin in the body. Along with a blend of phyto and marine proteins added to the extract to make it complete with all amino acids, its mission then becomes to regenerate and nourish aging and unhealthy cells bringing them back to their natural state (homeostasis). Laminine's Fibroblast Growth Factor (FGF) is largely responsible for this regeneration . Our body is incapable of producing its own FGF. We must get it from the food supply which is lacking today. Laminine is believed to be the only other known source of FGF. FGF reprograms adult stem cells and amino acids in the body to restore whatever part of the body that needs the most rehabilitation. Benefits seen with regular use of Laminine include (but are not limited to): stimulation of the body's natural DHEA to reduce physical and mental stress and support the adrenal system, increase in alertness and brain function, improvement in stamina and energy, quicker recovery after workouts, increase in muscle tone, more restful sleep, down-regulation of pain receptors in the body, increase in collagen for healthier skin, elevation of serotonin levels to raise mood, increase in libido, reduction in the signs of aging in general, and an overall sense of well-being. This supplement is well worth trying if you have fibromyalgia, blood sugar issues, heart disease, increased cholesterol levels, fatigue, or in menopause and currently not using hormones. Recommended dosing is two capsules per day for 15 days, then one capsule per day for maintenance. Laminine can be purchased from my office for $45/ thirty count** or online at: http://www.mylifepharm.com/judyponsford for $45.95/thirty count (no tax or shipping charges when ordering online). Click on the "order retail" link and fill in the information. Make sure to click the "update" link at the bottom of the page prior to submitting the order.

Testing:

Estronex^{sm} Profile: This is a 2 hydroxy/16 hydroxy estrogen ratio test. The ratio of "good to bad estrogens" can now be determined from a single urine specimen. This test will tell you whether or not your body is metabolizing its estrogens in the correct pathway. If you are interested in taking this simple urine test, please call my office for pricing and/or to order your kit.

Hormone Testing: Saliva testing is an accurate way to find out tissue hormone levels and where excess or deficiencies may exist. Prices vary for testing single and multiple hormones or for particular hormone kits according to each woman's particular station in life, such as premenopause, perimenopause, or postmenopause. Saliva testing is very reasonably priced compared to blood serum testing when paying out of pocket and well worth the money to help keep hormones in balance. Saliva testing is also an excellent way to assess adrenal function too. If you are interested in checking one or a number of your female or adrenal hormone levels, please call my office for pricing and/or to order your kit.

Thyroid Testing: If you are interested in more thorough thyroid testing, such as TSH, Free T3, Free T4, or rT3, please call my office for pricing and/or to order a thyroid panel or additional thyroid tests.

**Note: Any products that do not have a website for purchase may be purchased through my office at (303) 805-5466. Tax and shipping not included in price. Prices are subject to change.

If you have further questions about the products or testing I have suggested, you may direct your questions to my office by e-mail at: judyponsford@yahoo.com, or phone (303) 805-5466. I also carry several options for toxin-free skin care and weight loss.

Appendix II

Enzyme Therapy Test

Amylase Deficiency: If five or more of these characteristics apply to you, then you are amylase deficient.

___Yes ___No When you gain weight, it is evenly over the body, from your head to your feet.

___Yes ___No If you feel you are overweight, your excess fat is around the middle in the stomach and waist area. Men tend to have the "spare tire," while women hold fat in their buttocks.

___Yes ___No You have shoulders and hips that are the same width and usually in proportion to each other.

___Yes ___No You tend to crave simple carbs, such as desserts, breads, pastas, fruits, and vegetables.

___Yes ___No You are attracted to chocolate and coffee or caffeinated food or drinks.

___Yes ___No You lean toward depression or mood swings.

___Yes ___No You complain of cold hands and feet.

___Yes ___No If female, you have PMS.

___Yes ___No Your blood pressure is generally low.

___Yes ___No You have low blood sugar.

___Yes ___No Allergies are the norm for you.

Lipase Deficiency: If you answer yes to five or more of these statements, then you are lipase deficient.

___Yes ___No You have narrow shoulders and wider hips.

___Yes ___No If female, the larger part of your weight is in the buttocks and upper thighs.

___Yes ___No If male, your excess weight is in the abdomen.

___Yes ___No You crave tasty or strong-flavored dishes, such as spiced, creamed, salty, peppered, or smoked foods.

___Yes ___No You desire wine or a sweet beverage other than water with your meals.

___Yes ___No Your favorite desserts are rich, like ice cream or chocolate.

___Yes ___No You desire fried foods such as fish, chicken, onion rings, and French fries.

___Yes ___No You prefer Italian, Asian, and Mexican cuisines.

___Yes ___No You often suffer from indigestion.

___Yes ___No You have had gallbladder problems.

___Yes ___No You may be plagued by kidney and/or bladder infections.

___Yes ___No You have a tendency toward skin disorders, such as rashes or cysts.

Protease Deficiency: If five or more of these traits apply to you, then you are protease deficient.

___Yes ___No You carry your weight in your tummy and upper torso, including the back area.

___Yes ___No You have no shape to your buttocks (flat).

___Yes ___No Your legs are stout and firm, no matter what your age.

___Yes ___No You consider a meal complete only if it contains meat or some kind of protein.

___Yes ___No You tend to salt your food without tasting it first.

___Yes ___No You lean toward all proteins, such as lunch meats, sausage, fish, poultry, nuts, cheese, and eggs.

___Yes ___No You tend to suffer from stiff joints or pain in your left shoulder.

___Yes ___No You need to drink at least one beverage with your meal.

___Yes ___No You suffer from hypertension or high blood pressure.

___Yes ___No You feel more stressed than fatigued.

Lactase Deficiency: If you can answer yes to four or more of these questions, then you are lactase deficient.

___Yes ___No You tend to eat lots of dairy products.

___Yes ___No You gravitate to starchy foods and sweets.

___Yes ___No You enjoy dairy products but feel you have some sort of milk intolerance.

___Yes ___No Your body is the same size as when you were a teen. Your shape is somewhat boyish, wiry, or resembles having baby fat, but it has remained the same into maturity.

___Yes ___No You seemed to have matured later in life or you are the youngest-looking member in your family.

___Yes ___No You have ongoing intestinal problems, such as constipation, diarrhea, or a spastic colon.

___Yes ___No Your fat is distributed all over the body and feels soft. It is not just held in one area.

Appendix III

&

Yeast Questionnaire

___Yes ___No Retrieving knowledge from your parents or guardians, were you hospitalized as an infant?

___Yes ___No Retrieving knowledge from your parents or guardians, did you have chronic infections as a child, such as throat, ears, sinus, bronchial, or other severe infections from a bite, cut, or injury that required the use of antibiotics?

___Yes ___No As far back as *you* can remember, have you been plagued with chronic infections such as sinus, throat, ears, bladder, kidneys, or other?

___Yes ___No Have you ever been hospitalized?

___Yes ___No Have you ever taken prolonged courses of antibiotics (more than ten days)?

___Yes ___No Have you ever taken prolonged courses of steroids (inhalers included) for more than ten days?

___Yes ___No Have you been pregnant more than twice?

___Yes ___No If you have had children, did you have any C-section deliveries?

___Yes ___No Do you or have you ever taken synthetic hormones (including birth control pills)?

___Yes ___No Do you take any other synthetic medications, such as cholesterol or blood pressure meds?

___Yes ___No Do you take any over-the-counter medications on a regular basis, such as ibuprofen or sleep aids (other than herbals)?

___Yes ___No If you are taking hormones (bioidentical or synthetic), do you take estrogen only?

___Yes ___No Is your green food intake less than twice per day?

___Yes ___No Is your fruit/fiber intake less than once per day?

___Yes ___No Do you have fewer than two bowel movements per day?

___Yes ___No Do you drink alcohol (eight ounces or less) more than twice per week?

___Yes ___No Do you crave sweets?

___Yes ___No Is your diet high in simple carbohydrates, such as breads, potatoes, rice, sugary drinks, or high-carbohydrate health bars (combining all, more than two servings per day)?

___Yes ___No Are you bothered by fatigue, headaches, or depression?

___Yes ___No Do you have chemical sensitivities to things such as perfumes or other chemicals?

___Yes ___No Do you have food sensitivities?

___Yes ___No Do you have frequent vaginal infections?

___Yes ___No Do you have frequent bladder infections or been diagnosed with interstitial cystitis?

___Yes ___No Have you ever been diagnosed with endometriosis?

___Yes ___No Do you or have you suffered from infertility?

___Yes ___No Do you have digestive problems, such as bad breath, indigestion, constipation, gas, or bloating?

___Yes ___No Have you ever been diagnosed with an autoimmune disorder?

___Yes ___No Have you ever had a yeast or mold exposure?

___Yes ___No Have you ever been diagnosed with a skin disorder, such as psoriasis or eczema?

___Yes ___No Do you feel sick all over?

Please note that these questions are generalized questions and are not weighted. For instance, being on antibiotics or steroids for a long period of time would obviously carry more weight than not taking in enough daily fruit or fiber. However, this questionnaire is meant to give you an idea of what types of things would cause or point to systemic yeast and whether it is a mild, moderate, or severe problem.

If you answer *yes* to five or less of these questions, your yeast is mild, but your health would benefit from a yeast cleanse.

If you answer *yes* to six to ten of these questions, your yeast is moderate and a yeast cleanse is recommended to improve your overall general health.

If you answer *yes* to more than ten of these questions, your yeast is severe and clearing the yeast from your system is highly recommended so that your health does not continue to deteriorate.

Appendix IV

Progesterone to Estrogen Ratio from Serum Levels

To calculate your progesterone to estrogen ratio (P:E ratio), you must first make sure both the estrogen and progesterone are converted to the same weight units. Estrogen is reported in pg/ml (picograms per milliliter) while progesterone is reported in ng/ml (nanograms per milliliter). A simple math equation will allow you to do this.

Let's say that the level of your estradiol is 60 pg/ml and progesterone is 5.8 ng/ml. You need to convert the progesterone level to pg/ml so that it is in the same "weight unit" as the estrogen. Since there are 1000 picograms in each nanogram, you must multiply the progesterone level by 1000.

$5.8 \times 1000 = 5800$ pg/ml

Now you have progesterone in pg/ml, which you can compare to the estradiol.

Now you need to convert both to moles as the unit of weight (which just means molecules). The conversion looks like this:

Estradiol Conversion Factor: pg/ml x 3.671 = pMol/L

Progesterone Conversion Factor: pg/ml x 3.18 = pMol/L.

Now do the math:

Estradiol 60 pg/ml x 3.671 = 220.26

Progesterone 5800 pg/ml x 3.18 = 18444

Now divide progesterone by estradiol:

18444/220.26 = 83.73, so the **P:E = 84:1**

My Easy Quartile Analysis:

First Quartile: 20:1–50:1

Second Quartile: 51:1–100:1

Third Quartile: 101:1–150:1

Fourth Quartile: 151:1–200:1

According to my experience and if you are in the first quartile, you are most likely too low in progesterone and experiencing progesterone deficiency or estrogen dominance. I prefer that the P:E ratio fall at least in the second or third quartile (according to symptoms), which in this case it did. If the P:E falls in the fourth quartile, you probably will experience some insomnia or other symptoms of too much progesterone, as the P:E is most likely getting too high. Each woman is individual as to where she feels best, but this is a decent guideline for levels taken from blood serum.

Please note: you cannot compare blood serum hormone levels to saliva hormone levels. Blood serum levels are not tissue levels, so the comparison cannot be made.